9-15

W9-AGB-764

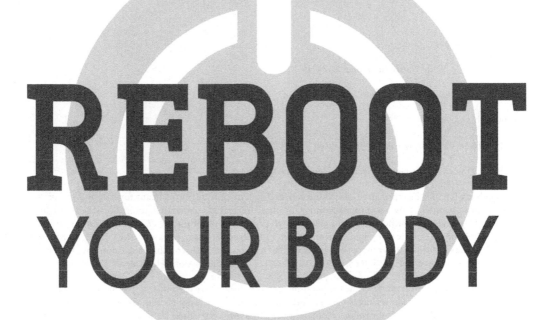

# REBOOT
## YOUR BODY

Unlocking the Genetic Secrets
to Permanent Weight Loss

## Rashelle Brown, BS, CPT, CHC

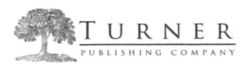

TURNER
PUBLISHING COMPANY

Turner Publishing Company

424 Church Street • Suite 2240 • Nashville, Tennessee 37219

445 Park Avenue • 9th Floor • New York, New York 10022

www.turnerpublishing.com

Reboot Your Body: Unlocking the Genetic Secrets to Permanent Weight Loss

Cover design: Mike Penticost

Book design: Mallory Perkins

Library of Congress Cataloging-in-Publication Data

Brown, Rashelle.
  Reboot your body : a step-by-step guide to permanent weight loss / by Rashelle Brown, BS, CPT, CHC.
     pages cm
  Includes bibliographical references.
  ISBN 978-1-63026-889-3 (pbk.)
1. Weight loss--Popular works. 2. Weight loss--Psychological aspects--Popular works. 3. Exercise--Popular works. 4. Food habits--Psychological aspects. 5. Self-care, Health--Popular works. I. Title.
  RM222.2.B7846 2015
  613.2'5--dc23
                     2015009482

Printed in the United States of America

15 16 17 18 19 20 10 9 8 7 6 5 4 3 2 1

My thanks to everyone who made this book possible, but especially to:

Garrison Keillor for encouraging me to write a weight loss book and for showing me, by example, the work ethic required of a successful writer; Alison Vandenberg, for giving me early advice that proved instrumental to the success of the book; my exceptional publicist, Gail Asche; Jennifer Rico of AideVantage for constructing the tables within the book; my agent, Anne Devlin, at Max Gartenberg Literary Agency; the entire editorial, marketing and publishing team at Turner Publishing; my mom for raising me to believe that I could do anything; and to Laura, who has been a constant source of support and who believed in me when belief was in short supply.

# CONTENTS

## Introduction

# WHAT'S DIFFERENT THIS TIME?

You're reading this book because you want to lose weight and nothing you've tried has stuck. Chances are, you've tried many times before—sometimes making no progress at all, other times losing the weight but always eventually gaining it back. You've dieted, exercised, or attended weight-loss classes—maybe you've tried all three. So what could be different this time? What could this book possibly tell you that all the others have missed? Well, quite honestly, a lot.

This is not a diet book or an exercise program. It doesn't tell you to stop eating wheat or start eating like a cave dweller. It doesn't promise that you'll look just like that celebrity fitness trainer or that you can eat all you want and magically lose weight. This book is not based on a quick solution or an attractive lie you might be eager to believe.

*This book is about you.*

More precisely, it's about finding a unique and specific solution to achieve permanent weight loss based on your physical and emotional makeup. This book offers you a step-by-step guide to finally finding the right combination of diet, exercise, and behavior changes that will work with your body and, more importantly, with your personality.

*Based on cutting-edge science, this book will show you how*
*implementing new patterns of behavior can rewire your physical makeup.*

It's not just about changing your eating and exercise habits to result in more calories burned than consumed. The key is that my approach will change the way your body responds to food *permanently*. Ultimately, your success hinges on learning to harness the power of habit in order to rewire your mind, which in turn will permanently change your body.

It may seem odd that a personal trainer has written a weight-loss book that places more emphasis on the mind than on the body, but let me explain why I've done so.

For a very long time, I couldn't understand why weight-loss studies always had such dismal outcomes, regardless of the factors manipulated or methods employed. If people dieted, they lost a little weight; if people exercised, they lost a little weight; if they did both, they lost a little more weight. But eventually, the vast majority of subjects put the weight back on. It was very disheartening to me, as I was looking for a standardized "formula" that I could use to help my clients be their best selves.

One day, while reading a more detailed study, I was excited to find that some of the subjects had lost a great deal of weight, and more importantly, they were able to keep the weight off through the eighteen-month follow-up period. But my excitement was confounded when I learned that even this thorough and well-written study couldn't conclude (with any certainty) *why* some subjects enjoyed success while others did not. At that point it seemed futile to search for answers that could help my individual clients from studies that only looked at the average outcomes across a group of subjects. None of the studies I'd read could offer any insight into what might make a particular individual lose weight permanently. As I pored over the criteria the scientists had used, hunting for some clue, an idea struck me: if the key could not be found in what the researchers were measuring, then it must be among those things they were ignoring.

In all of the high-quality weight-loss studies I'd read, the primary variables manipulated (diet, exercise, medication) were different for each one, but the control variables—the "outlying factors" they used to weed out potentially corrupted data—were very similar. The studies all very smartly accounted for things like age, gender, family health history, certain genetic conditions and disorders, the presence or history of disease, whether the subject smoked, current level of fitness, and so on. But at that moment, I realized those factors were all *physical*—none of them were *mental*, *emotional*, or *behavioral*.

For the first time in a long time, I got excited. Certainly the difference among personalities, lifestyle habits, and other behavioral characteristics must at least partially explain the widely varying results among a group of participants who had been selected *for* their physical similarities. It seemed highly plausible that these nonphysical characteristics were responsible for putting certain people into the successful group while the others were left out.

It's true that we each have a unique physical makeup. But don't we also each have a personality that is entirely unique? How then can we discount this whole host of "outlying factors" when trying to determine what methods might be most effective for weight loss, or any other endeavor for that matter?

Incorporating these "outlying factors" into a new approach, I immediately redirected my studies, expanding my reading and research to give me better insight into how I could help my clients reach their goals and ultimately change their lives. A whole other realm of scientific, medical, and psychological research opened up to me once I knew what I was looking for.

I was surprised to find that this research had been going on for decades. I wondered why I hadn't heard much about it in the mainstream media. Nearly every day you can find an article online or in print discussing the merits of this diet, that workout, or a promising new weight-loss drug. After reading more, I suspected that the reason I hadn't heard much about these other fields yet had to do with money.

There was a recurring theme in everything I previously had been reading. Each of the studies was narrowly focused on proving that X hormone or Y gene was responsible for a certain function related to obesity. The researchers were (and still are) all racing to find a substance or therapy that could influence those genetic and hormonal factors, bringing an end to obesity. If the day ever arrives when a pharmaceutical company is able to do this, we will all celebrate, and that pharmaceutical company may end up ruling the world. But the crazy part is that the mechanisms for controlling those hormonal and genetic factors already exist within you! You already possess everything you need to successfully lose weight and keep it off. There's not much money wrapped up in this solution, so the funding for studies is sparse and there is no mainstream marketing associated with it. You can spend a few bucks on a book like this or do your own research at little or no cost, but apart from that, there are no products to sell, no ads to run, and no big sponsorships to net. The government isn't subsidizing behavior change; it's subsidizing food and drugs. The "formula" I had been looking for was there all along, and it's actually pretty simple:

*By changing your behaviors, you create new neural pathways in your brain; those new neural pathways translate into habits; if those habits are kept up over time they result in lifestyle changes; and these changes in lifestyle transform your body's physiological mechanisms at the cellular level, rewiring your body for good.*

There are no gimmicks, no prepackaged food or protein shakes, no drugs, and no crazy fad workouts. Of course, the idea of using behavior change to lose weight is nothing new. The new part is finally finding the right combination of behaviors and skills that will work with *your* personality and *your* genetic makeup, and creating an environment that supports those changes forever.

As I read books and position papers, research abstracts and full studies, I began to understand how much control the mind really has over the physical body. I also learned that because of the highly adaptive nature of the human body, the way your body reacts and responds to things today can be vastly different from how it will react just a few short months from now.

The fascinating fields of neuroscience and epigenetics (literally translated "above genetics") are beginning to prove that, even though you might not have inherited an ideal set of genes, you have much more control than you think over which of those genes are *expressed* and which are instead *suppressed*. In short:

> *By manipulating certain factors within your control repeatedly over time, you can actually turn certain genes on or off.*[1]

This, in turn, can change many things about you, like whether you will contract a certain disease or whether you will remain overweight.

This might all sound like weird science, but epigenetic research applied to cancer studies has been going on for decades. Long before the mapping of the human genome was complete, scientists were studying external environmental factors and the mutation of genes. It has only been in the past decade, however, that these studies began focusing on obesity. I first encountered the term *epigenetics* during a continuing education seminar taught by PhD exercise physiologist Mark Kelly.[2] His seminar really sparked my current line of research and changed the way I was working with overweight clients.

I can't blame you if you still feel a little skeptical, though. This is relatively new science, and it can sound a bit more like science fiction at times. But I think it's very likely that within the next five to ten years, epigenetic research will begin to have major implications on the weight-loss market, so that finally even the mainstream media will begin to take notice.

Because I'm not a neuroscientist or a geneticist, and presumably you aren't either, let me explain my practical understanding of how this all works by giving you a personal example.

## I'm Not the Person I Used to Be

There's a reason why I can consistently eat many more calories than most of my overweight clients yet maintain my current weight while my clients struggle to shed a pound or two here or there. It is true that most of my calories are fairly healthy ones, and that I'm a pretty active person, but many of my clients weigh twice what I do and spend nearly the same amount of time exercising. So, even if I exercise quite a bit harder than they do, theoretically we should burn around the same number of calories each day. And yet I am eating several hundred or even a thousand more calories than they are, every single day.

"Ah, it's your metabolism!" you might say. And you'd be right, my metabolism is running higher than theirs. But the thing is, my metabolism *shouldn't* be higher than theirs. There is a problem with the "formula" here: Body weight is the largest factor affecting energy expenditure (given similar activity levels). If a 200-pound person and I do the same activity—walk three miles briskly, for example—the 200-pound person will burn nearly 50 percent more calories per minute than I will.

Even when adjusting for fat versus fat-free body mass, the numbers don't add up. If I weigh 135 pounds at 20 percent body fat, my fat-free mass is around 108 pounds. But if my client weighs 200 pounds at 35 percent body fat, his fat-free mass is around 130 pounds. So even though a larger *percentage* of my body weight is fat-free mass, my client still has 20 percent more fat-free mass than I do. Thus, he should be burning many more calories than I am *all of the time*.

There's something much deeper going on that's making this crucial difference between me and my clients: my body *knows* that I am thin and fit, while my client's body knows that he is fat. My body knows this because my brain knows it, and I'm not talking about my conscious, reasoning brain. I mean that other part of the brain—the subconscious brain, or the *mind*.

You're probably feeling really skeptical right about now. Or maybe you're a little intrigued. If you're the adventurous type, perhaps you feel a tingle of excitement. Let me give you a few examples of how what the mind knows (or *thinks it knows*) can cause amazing physical outcomes.

Scattered across southern Appalachia, there are Pentecostal devotees who periodically participate in faith rituals in which they handle poisonous rattlesnakes (often getting bitten) and even drink strychnine, so strong is their belief that the Lord will protect them. And overwhelmingly, these individuals meet no ill fate.[3] There are any number of reasons why this may be, from the physical well-being of the snakes to the level of experience of the handlers; but while those factors vary among churches and snakes, what is constant throughout is the deeply held belief among handlers that they will be protected.

Now let's shift from religion to science. For decades, psychologists and psychiatrists have been documenting significant physiological changes in individuals diagnosed with Dissociative Identity Disorder (formerly Multiple Personality Disorder). Things like visual acuity, colorblindness, allergic reactions, rashes, and even scars have been clinically observed to change, disappear, and reappear in the span of time it takes the patient to transition from one personality to another, because the patient's mind *believes* that he or she is a different person entirely.[4]

A little less fantastic is the research surrounding the placebo effect. Strong evidence gathered in studies spanning more than two hundred years and across a variety of fields of medical study suggest that a placebo is likely to produce favorable outcomes similar to the drug or other therapy being tested 30 percent (or more) of the time.[5] This means that people *experience physiological changes simply because they believe* they have been administered a drug or received a therapy or surgery, when in fact they have not.[6]

These are some pretty convincing examples of the kind of power that the mind can have over the physical body, but how can this make a difference with something like weight loss? After all, it's accepted as fact that weight loss simply comes down to more calories expended than consumed—and yet we see examples of huge deviations from this "rule" everywhere around us.

Don't we all know at least one person who can seemingly eat whatever they want and not gain weight? And don't we also know plenty of people who are faithfully dieting and exercising month in and month out with little or no progress? Well, epigenetics tells us that the difference between these two types of people has as much to do with the electrical and chemical signals their brains are sending to their bodies' cells as it has to do with the genetic makeup of those cells.

*Your brain can be rewired to control your body in favorable ways,
regardless of your genetic predisposition to be fat or thin.*[7]

Here's an oversimplified example of how it works: When I eat a big dinner, wash it down with my favorite beer, and finish it off with a piece of pie, my brain perceives this huge influx of calories and says, "Oh good—more fuel! We need to burn this!" But when my overweight friend sitting across the table from me eats the same exact meal, his brain perceives this huge influx of calories and says, "Oh good—more fuel! We need to store this!" Because my brain knows that I am fit and thin, and his brain knows that he is fat, they each act accordingly, sending out instructions to the rest of the body to either burn those calories as fuel now or to store them as fat, in case they need to be converted back into fuel during a later "energy crisis" that will likely never come. A simple way to think of differences in metabolism, then, is to consider what two different bodies will do with the same number and type of calories.

The great news for you is that I'm living proof of a weight-loss success story. For years and years I struggled with weight, failing miserably to shed even five pounds, growing steadily heavier and more miserable. The tipping point came for me when I failed to "make weight" during a routine weigh-in when I was in the military, and I was in jeopardy of being put on what was so delicately dubbed "the fat boy program."

I got desperate and starved myself for a week and squeaked in under my maximum at my next weigh-in, but I knew that I had to change things in a big way or I'd find myself in the same situation six months down the road. What followed was a long, erratic, and arduous process that ultimately resulted in my losing 30 pounds over two years. Ten years later, having learned a lot, I finally dropped the last 10 pounds, and have been at my ideal weight ever since.

Of course, you don't want to wait ten or twelve years to reach your ideal weight, and you don't have to! This book is the result of my hard-won knowledge and experience. It is a step-by-step guide that *will* transform you from the physical person you are now to the one you dream of becoming. If you follow the steps and do the work, I promise you will feel rebooted.

## How to Use This Book

Using this book to achieve your goals is simple: get a notebook and a pen, and work your way through the pages step-by-step. If you're tech savvy and always have your smart phone or mobile device with you, then any electronic notebook app will do, but a standard spiral-bound, lined notebook you can pick up for under two bucks at the drug store may actually work even better.

When you get to an exercise that requires you to write something down, it will be indicated by the pen icon you see above. That will be your cue that there's work to be done, so be prepared to devote the required amount of time to it. It's important that you take your time and put real effort into each exercise, and not skip over any of them. The order of the steps and exercises in this book are the key to the high rate of success among a broad range of clients I have worked with. By following along and working diligently, you can create a program that will work for you. To help you out, I've included character examples for each exercise. I've pulled these examples from the real-world experiences of my clients. (Of course, the names have been changed!)

## Prologue

# HOW DID WE GET INTO THIS MESS?

L et's back up for just a minute and get a sense of how and why you've been caught up in this overweight epidemic in the first place. Understanding some of the forces that are acting against you will help you later on when it's time to start thinking about how you'll defeat them.

If you live in America and have been paying attention at all, you have undoubtedly heard some of the following statistics:

- From 1960 to 2010, the percentage of obese adults in the United States nearly tripled.[1]
- Over two-thirds of the adult population in the United States is now overweight or obese.[2]
- Currently, one in every three Americans are likely to be diagnosed with type 2 diabetes at some point in his or her lifetime.[3]
- Obesity is the number two cause of preventable death in the United States and likely to soon overtake smoking for the top spot.[4]
- *For the first time ever, there is a good chance that a child born today will have a shorter life expectancy than his or her parents due to lifestyle-related factors.*[5]

Indeed, there seems to be no end to the bad-news health headlines in the media these days. And what's worse than the headlines, numbers, charts, and graphs is that behind each and every tic on a scientist's stat sheet there is a real person living a life worse than the one they could be living. Chances are, it's a person who is just like someone you know, someone you love, or maybe just like you. And the most discouraging factor of all is that it's preventable—we are doing this to ourselves!

During World War II, a primary problem facing the military was that too many recruits were underweight. Today, the US military turns down one in four applicants because they are too heavy.[6] And, representative of the US population in general, 64 percent of *active duty* military members were either overweight or obese in 2011.[7]

So, over the course of one lifetime, our nation has gone from having scarcely enough to feed its fighting men to having to turn young volunteers away and placing thousands of active duty members on probationary programs because of their weight. How has this happened?

The collective woes of the nation can be viewed in conjunction with the more intimate factors at play for almost any obese individual. To put it plainly, there are a host of reasons why any one person becomes overweight, and those reasons tend to be very similar among all Americans. Let's take a look at those biological, social, and environmental factors that have led us to where we are today.

## A Very Brief History of the (Dietary) Evolution of Man

For the ten-thousand-year period leading up to the 1900s, human living conditions changed very little and very slowly. The effort and energy required to keep ourselves alive took up most of our waking hours. The procurement of shelter, clean water, and food were pretty much all our ancestors had time to think about. Leisure time was more or less limited to those few fleeting moments after the sun went down and before they dropped onto their cave floors or into their straw-filled beds, exhausted from the day's work.

For thousands of years, man's diet was local and seasonal to the extreme. The idea of eating a food that had been grown or procured more than a day's walk away was preposterous, if even conceivable.

Even after roads and aqueducts were created, there was rarely an abundance of food. The domestication of beasts of burden allowed for the tiniest bit more variety in the types of food a tribe or village had access to, and it also made non-communal living possible, allowing families or individuals to be a bit farther from the central water and food supply. But it was still largely up to each family or tribe to provide for themselves, and farming and hunting methods were primitive and inefficient. Later our ability to build seaworthy vessels and navigate the oceans caused the next big leap forward in large-scale trade as food and other supplies were brought in from sources much farther away.

As transportation modes got better and trade continued to flourish, food became a commodity, rather than just a bare necessity. People now had some degree of choice about what they ate (or at least those in the upper echelons of society did). But then there was a long period of time in which little changed. For several hundred years, ships and horses were the primary means of transportation, until the early nineteenth century when the locomotive steam engine was invented and put into wide use, solidifying the industrial revolution here in the United States. This was a real game changer! Large quantities of all manner of goods could now be hauled across land, drastically cutting the amount of time those goods spent in transit, making a great diversity of foods available across various regions of the country. More and more settlements began popping up all over the country, not just near major sea ports or other large bodies of water.

The thing that really revolutionized our food supply (and therefore our diets), though, was the commercial drilling and production of petroleum in conjunction with the mass-production of the internal combustion engine. By 1925, it was possible for a farmer using a gasoline-powered tractor to produce an acre of wheat in five worker-hours—less than one-tenth the time it took to produce the same acre in 1800.[8]

During the World Wars, scientists developed ways to mass-produce and package meals for soldiers. Thus, packaged food was born! After World War II ended, the men returned home from war and agricultural production returned to—and then surpassed—previous levels.

Growing right alongside the agricultural boom was unprecedented scientific work in the food industry. New discoveries made it possible to grow more food using fewer resources, to make the food look and taste more appealing, and to give it a much longer shelf life. So there was a kind of "perfect storm" brewing, in which our country was able to utilize defunct war facilities and create jobs for its citizens by refitting them as new factories that processed and packaged an amount and variety of food that was previously unimagined. Together, these new technologies and delivery systems grew the food supply and its processing and distribution exponentially over the next several decades.

For post-war Americans, I'm sure it truly seemed to be a golden age. The amount of time and effort it took women to prepare the family's meals was drastically reduced, giving them the opportunity to consider working outside the home for their own personal and financial benefit, rather than out of necessity for the war effort.

And so, we cooked less and we ate more. We ate these new foods, and the government began subsidizing big agriculture, telling farmers to "Get big or Get out!"[9] So farms got bigger, and by the 1970s, we were producing enough food for our own country plus $20 billion in exports with an agricultural labor force that comprised only 4.6 percent of the working population at that time.[10] We had learned how to use machinery, chemicals, and mass-production to feed an entire nation cheaply, quickly, and conveniently.

But biologically, we had no time to adjust to these new living conditions. Our bodies did not suddenly develop a new kind of energy system to handle all of this new food. Where we had previously been walking behind a team of mules to plow up the earth by hand and plant a crop that might or might not feed one family for one season, we were now handed complete meals in tin-wrapped containers, which we could quickly cook in our new electric ovens. We no longer had to chop wood, build fires, carry water, and boil it before drinking, cleaning, or cooking. We could hunt for pleasure or to supplement our already resplendent food supply, or we could choose not to hunt at all. Instead, we could stay home and be entertained by this new thing called the television.

Between prepackaged TV dinners, an abundant food supply, and decreased daily labor, it's easy to see why we began to grow fat. Our food systems and our labor mechanisms progressed far more rapidly than our biological systems possibly could. We were presented with far more food, which required far less work (and therefore energy) to procure and prepare, and we happily said, "Yes, thank you!"

But if we look at the issue more closely, we can see a few other reasons why the obesity epidemic has spiraled out of control so quickly. Beyond the purely biological and technological contributors, there are other factors having to do with money, politics, and basic human nature. The three work together, creating the powerful forces that act upon you every day, making you want to eat larger quantities of foods that are low in nutritional quality.

## Someone Is Getting Rich While You Are Getting Fat

Today, Americans spend about $40 billion annually on diet products and weight-loss programs.[11] And we spend $117 billion or more annually on fast food.[12] Nestle reported over $7 billion in world-wide candy bar sales in 2013,[13] and nearly $12 billion in revenues under its "Nutrition and HealthCare" enterprise in that same year (Nestle owns the Lean Cuisine frozen entrée and Boost nutritional beverage brands).[14] Meanwhile, in 2012, Americans spent $176 billion on direct medical costs for the treatment of diabetes, just one of the diseases closely tied to obesity.[15]

What makes us spend all that money? Marketing, of course! In 2008, there were nearly thirty-five thousand food and beverage brand commercials aired during prime-time television—that's about ninety-five per evening.[16] You can't attend a movie, a concert, a play, or a little league game anywhere in this country without being offered food or beverages for sale. Sales of snacks and beverages from vending machines in schools alone average $2.3 billion per year. A high school can net as much as $30,000 annually by offering this junk to your kids.[17]

Think about your average day for a moment. How many times do you think you are marketed to by the food and beverage industry? How many times do you drive or walk past a restaurant with eye-popping advertising marquis? How many food and drink commercials do you see on television, read in magazines, newspapers, or on billboards, or hear on the radio? How many coupons do you get in the mail or on the food products you purchase?

Food is everywhere, and more often than not it's the high-sugar, high-fat, ready-to-go stuff because it's the cheapest to make and the easiest to sell. By now, our taste buds have been programmed to crave the stuff. Add the typical busy American schedule into the mix, and the conditions are ripe for unhealthy eating. We're tired, we're hungry, and we don't have time to shop and cook. Then we see and smell this quick and easy option, and we're tempted. We cave in and bring home this food-that's-not-food to serve to our families. A short time later, we collapse on the couch, our energy sapped, our resolve near zero, and we subject ourselves to more marketing from the industry, increasing the chances that we will get up tomorrow and do it all over again.

So what can we do about it?

## Move to the Head of the Class

After reading all of that, you might be smiling and thinking, "I knew this wasn't my fault! It's all that other stuff that got me to this unhealthy place." And it's true that these historical, environmental, and social factors *have* played a big role in our obesity epidemic. But of course, these factors alone do not represent the reason why you and 1.4 billion other people across the globe are overweight.[18]

*You are overweight because you*
*eat too much and move too little.*

You might be drawing a breath to protest right now, and I'm guessing that you might want to bring up a couple of *other* contributing factors. I can hear you asking, "What about my thyroid? My metabolism? Everyone in my family is overweight—what about those *genetics* you keep mentioning?"

This is an area frequently studied and widely debated across many disciplines in medical research. Fortunately, recent findings in the field of epigenetics render it something of a moot point. While the old science[19] argued that inherited genes could account for as much as 75 percent of the tendency to become obese, the new science[20] has demonstrated that genetic makeup is far less important than genetic expression. The fact that you possess the "fat gene"—if one does exist (the scientists are still duking it out over this one)—will only make you fat if you engage in the behaviors that cause its expression. In other words, by living the right kind of lifestyle your genetic predisposition toward obesity can be suppressed.

Your genetic makeup is over 99 percent identical to every other human on earth, and the human genome has not changed much at all over the past sixty years.[21] What *has* changed dramatically in that time, however, is our food culture. It's not that our bodies are suddenly trying to hold on to every calorie we consume, but rather that we are consuming more calories than we have at any other time in history.

Unless you suffer from one of a few very rare conditions, you are overweight because of the lifestyle you've been living up to now, irrespective of your inherited genes. Don't feel bad about this, though; in fact, it should come as very good news to you—because *those are the factors you can control*! In this book I'll teach you how to use lifestyle habits to manipulate your genes and change your body. It's not the sort of thing that will put your weight-loss effort on autopilot, but it will finally put you on a level playing field.

At the end of the day, despite your genes, the way you were raised, the changes in the food industry, and all of the millions of dollars of persuasive marketing out there, *you are a sentient being capable of exercising free will*, and your current physical condition is the result of millions of decisions you have made over the space of days, weeks, months, and years. These decisions have carved out well-traveled synaptic highways in your brain, prompting cravings and setting your eating behaviors on autopilot. Your first order of business is to stop traveling on those destructive highways and start carving out new roads.

*What this all boils down to, really,
is learning to make better decisions.*

I'd love to tell you that this will be easy, but unfortunately, the numbers are stacked against you. Research has shown that only around 20 percent of people who lose a significant amount of weight are able to keep it off for one year or more.[22] That's a pretty low success rate considering how many people have tried and continue to try losing weight. Knowing this forces you to make a decision right now. Will you lament your slim chances and begin your weight-loss effort expecting to fail? Or will you turn your focus instead toward what it will take to get you to the head of the class? How can you be among the successful 20 percent?

Read on to gather the information and tools you'll need to do just that. What follows is a systematic approach that will lead you to weight-loss success. I want to stress at the outset, however, that this is an *active process*—there are no shortcuts, magic pills, diets, or workouts that will quickly and permanently strip away the pounds you have spent years putting on. This will be hard work, and it will be a relatively long process.

Changing your body's genetic expression only happens as the result of sustained behaviors practiced over time. Fortunately, many of those behaviors will also result in daily calorie deficits, leading to short-term weight loss, so you'll start making progress toward your weight-loss goal right away. This book, unlike so many weight-loss gimmicks, will help you construct and follow a detailed personal plan that will turn that small, short-term progress into a life-altering, permanent goal achievement. So come on, let's get started!

# Part One:

# YOUR STRUCTURAL ROADMAP TO
# PERMANENT WEIGHT LOSS

Obesity is all in your head. Think about it: Your brain controls *every* function in your body, down to the most basic cellular level. It does so by using a sophisticated system of communication that involves hormones, chemicals, and electrical signals. Regardless of which part of the brain is called upon or which method of delivery it employs, it controls the body's systems based on what it perceives as the current environmental conditions. But apart from the very limited sensory input it gets from your immediate surroundings, your brain doesn't actually *know* what those conditions are. Rather, it makes an educated guess based on your body's biological *history*.

Some of this history is way in the past—like ten million years ago. This history is stored in the "reptilian" part of your brain that controls automatic reflex responses and life-sustaining biological functions like breathing. Only millions of additional years of evolution can make changes to this part of the brain. But the other parts of your brain are much newer and more sophisticated, and most of that biological history comes from the *experiences of your life since birth*. You can think of this history as the information your brain uses as the blueprint for running your body.

So, if you've been overweight since you were a young child, or even if you *thought* you were overweight, or *were told* that you were overweight, your brain has a lot of history saying, "Hey, my body is fat. I need to keep it that way, because that's what I know." And your rational brain can try all it wants to convince the subconscious brain that it doesn't want your body to be fat, but until the subconscious brain *learns* that your body is not fat, then systems and signals from your brain will function as they always have.

In 2008, Dr. Dean Ornish and his colleagues conducted ground-breaking research demonstrating that lifestyle changes altered gene expression in cancer patients.[1] Many studies prior to this had shown that poor lifestyle habits caused negative mutations of certain genes, but the Ornish research was the first to show that the opposite could also be true: by improving certain lifestyle factors (diet, exercise, and stress management), the genes responsible for a number of conditions and pathologies (cancer, heart disease, diabetes, and obesity) could be *suppressed*, halting or even reversing those conditions.[2] Since 2008, other epigenetic studies have confirmed that diet and exercise can change the way the body metabolizes and stores fat.[3]

Think back to my earlier example comparing me to my obese client. According to the charts and calculators, we have similar total daily caloric expenditures, but on average, I routinely take in many more calories. It makes sense, then, that my body is expressing certain genes that keep my metabolism running high, burning calories at a high rate, while my client's body is expressing certain other genes that are doing just the opposite. The repetitive practice of my healthy habits has carved out specific neural pathways, so that the nature of the signals my brain is sending are different from those my client's brain is sending.[4] This means that it's easier for me to resist food and beverage cravings, I am more likely to exercise every day, and healthy foods taste even better to me. In other words, I am operating on a kind of positive feedback loop that makes my weight maintenance efforts much easier than those of my overweight clients. All of this is the result of my brain's biological history, which I have been carefully writing with the daily behaviors and habits that make up my lifestyle. For years I've been practicing certain habits that have caused my body to *know* that I am a fit, thin individual and to respond accordingly.

Now, does this mean that I can eat a big dinner, wash it down with my favorite beer, and finish it off with a piece of pie every night and never gain weight? Of course not! The key factor here is that my healthy habits are *ongoing*. When I have a string of days where I've strayed from my good habits, the scale does start to creep up. But I am far from a perfect eater, and I do indulge more often than a woman of my age, height, and weight metabolically "should" be able to. The epigenetic advantage I'm talking about is a percentage difference, not an order of magnitude. No one can get to a state where they can eat cheeseburgers and pizza every day and not gain weight unless they're compensating for it with hours of vigorous daily activity. But by finding the life-style habits that are uniquely best for you, you *can* get to the place where you'll finally start seeing your weight-loss efforts pay off in a big and permanent way.

Our bodies are in a constant state of adaptation. Our stress levels, sleep patterns, nutrition, and activity are never the same from one day to the next; we are exposed to either more or fewer harmful toxins; we consume more or less of our drugs of choice; we are sick or well, injured or healthy. And yet our bodies function in basically the same manner, day after day, until one or a few of these factors change *and* that change is maintained for a relatively long stretch of time. For example, you drink a beer a day and you probably don't feel much effect, but when you have two beers, you get a little tipsy. But if you start drinking two beers a day, pretty soon you will feel just like you used to when you drank only one.

Similarly, studies on caffeine consumption and athletic performance have all shown a positive correlation: When consumed at a certain level so many minutes before an event, caffeine helps most athletes perform better than they would under similar conditions without the drug. However, there is *no effect at all* if the athlete regularly consumes caffeine because his or her body has already adapted to it. We commonly refer to this phenomenon as "tolerance." Simply put, your body "learns" new things at the cellular level all the time based on what you expose it to repeatedly, or based on the *biological history* you are creating. It also means that starting right now, you can get your body out of its current state of homeostasis—you can unstick your metabolism! The trick is that you have to employ the proper techniques, and you have to keep them up over time. And then, when your body is used to that, if you want to change more, you'll have to teach it something new again.

## The Simple Solution: Weight Loss Starts with Your Way of Thinking

Ultimately, what leads to significant and lasting weight loss is a change in your calorie balance: taking in fewer calories (and higher-quality ones, please) than your body burns. That's the part you've always known but have never been able to successfully implement on a permanent basis. What you might not have known is that

*You can be successful this time,*
*no matter how many times you have failed before!*

While the basic formula for weight loss is simple and universal, we have to find the way to effectively implement it so that it works for *you*. There cannot possibly be a weight-loss "program" that works the same way for a multitude of different people. There are thousands of variables at play making your specific situation unique only to you. In terms of actually shedding the pounds, the most important of those variables are physical—your current physical condition, your predisposition to certain injuries and diseases, your usual level of activity, the way you normally eat, the way your metabolism is currently functioning, and, don't forget, your genetic makeup. All of these things determine your body's unique physical characteristics. The only way to alter them is to rewrite your biological history, and doing that starts with rewiring your brain.

Your brain will need to start sending out chemical and electrical messages along new pathways, and the only way to carve out those pathways is through sustained behavior modification. Behavior change is hard, though, right? So I'm giving you a clear roadmap for how to proceed, and plenty of proven techniques that you can use to tip the scale in your favor. While the steps and exercises in this book are the same for everyone, the work you'll do to complete each one should be entirely tailored to you. It will be a fact-finding exploration of who you are, how you operate physically, mentally, and emotionally, and ultimately of who you want to be.

## Chapter One

# LAYING THE FOUNDATION FOR SUCCESS

Before you can start thinking about the individual behaviors you want to change, you'll need to do some background work. More than anything, this process is one of self-discovery and self-honesty. It requires you to ask yourself tough questions and to not be content with the usual, easy answers. It means taking responsibility, making compromises, and at times, letting go of certain parts of yourself. That can be difficult and painful, but it's necessary if you are truly committed to making a lifestyle change. I told you in the introduction that this is not a diet or exercise book. It doesn't make false claims or promise an easy transformation. Instead, it gives you the honest answer to the question: "How can I finally lose the weight and keep it off?" The first part of that answer requires telling yourself exactly how you got here in the first place.

## Step One:
## STATE THE PROBLEM

### What's *Really* Wrong?

It's tempting to make this an obvious, one-sentence answer: "The problem is that I'm overweight." But, as with every exercise in this book, you will need to be as specific as possible when completing it. A one-sentence answer won't give you any insight. Dig deeper and fill those blank lines on the first page of your notebook. Try to really get at the heart of what's going on with you. This exercise begins to form your motivation for embarking on your weight-loss journey. It tells you why you're even considering this long and difficult process in the first place. It puts you face-to-face with all of those uncomfortable facts you've been trying hard to ignore for so long. It may be the first bit of open, honest communication you've had with yourself in a very long time.

##  Exercise 1: State the Problem.

Be specific. How overweight are you? What problems is your weight creating for your health, happiness, relationships, or career? How long has this been a problem, and when did it start? Don't get into the specific things that *caused* your weight gain (that will be addressed in a later exercise). In this exercise, I want you to write about all of the ways that your current physical condition is keeping you from living the life you want.

## Character Example

Bob is forty-three years old, six feet two inches tall, weighs 358 pounds, and has recently been diagnosed with type 2 diabetes and moderate to serious atherosclerosis. Bob's doctor has told him that if he doesn't lose some weight and become more active, he'll be putting himself at great risk. His doctor has recommended that Bob start by trying to lose 10 percent of his current body weight over the next six months. Bob fills the first page of his notebook with the following journal entry:

*Exercise 1: State the Problem.*

*I am forty-three years old and more than 140 pounds overweight. I've just been diagnosed with type 2 diabetes and told by my doctor that my coronary arteries are about 30 to 40 percent blocked. I was sent home with a handful of prescriptions and advised to do "whatever it takes" to lose some weight. My doctor said that, to start, I should aim to lose about 35 to 40 pounds. This seems like a drop in the bucket, but I guess I have to start somewhere.*

*My weight has been an issue for me since the year after I graduated from college and quit playing football. In my late twenties, whenever I gained a bunch of weight, I could lose it again pretty easily, but each time that happened, I kept on three to five extra pounds, so by the time I hit thirty, I was up about 40 pounds from what had been a somewhat bulky 215. From there, things just got worse. I found it harder and harder to lose the weight, and on my fortieth birthday, I weighed in at just under 298 pounds. I was determined that I was going to lose 100 pounds, and for a few months, things went pretty well. Then I started having knee pain and I couldn't work out anymore. My progress stopped and I got frustrated and gave up, and I've been in a losing battle with every fad diet that has hit the market ever since. The result has been a disastrous cycle of failure and depression, and I've GAINED another 60 pounds!*

*I know that if I don't change my ways and lose a massive amount of weight, I might not live to see my fiftieth birthday, or maybe even my forty-fifth.*

*My weight negatively impacts my life in nearly every way. I don't sleep well because I have weight-related sleep apnea. It's hard to find clothes that fit me, so I'm limited in my wardrobe. This (along with the fact that I am just plain fat) makes it hard for me to look professional and be taken seriously by clients, peers, and managers at work. I know my weight has negatively impacted my career. I'm unable to do a lot of the things my family enjoys—I can't play ball with my son for more than a few minutes without feeling like I'm going to keel over, I can't make it more than a block with my wife, who goes for a walk after dinner nearly every night, and my days of camping are over— there is no way that I can sleep on an air mattress or fit onto any standard cot. I miss the outdoors and am tired of living a life that is so limited by my weight.*

## Step Two:
# DECIDE THAT YOU *WANT* TO LOSE WEIGHT AND *BELIEVE* THAT YOU WILL

### It's Your Prerogative to Change Your Mind

Changing your weight-related behaviors starts with reframing the way you think. Your thoughts and attitudes constitute your beliefs. Beliefs trigger behaviors, and behaviors become habits. That's the part you might already know, and it's the basic premise behind every sensible weight-loss program. But changing your thinking also has the potential to do something much more important. When sustained over the long term, this new thinking gets into your brain "above genetics," redrawing the blueprint your brain uses to tell your body how to behave. So if you want to change not only your habits but your physiological mechanisms as well, the first thing you need to do is change your frame of mind. And that doesn't involve just changing your thoughts; it means changing your *deepest beliefs* about who you are. This is real work that you must do diligently, consistently, and daily. You can begin this work right now, by deciding that you *want* to lose weight and *believing* that you will.

## Do You Want to Lose Weight?

The answer to this would seem obvious because you are reading this book. But take a moment and consider what I'm asking: Knowing that you're embarking on a months-long process of self-examination and hard work, is the desired end-goal *truly* worth it to you? Are you ready to change the person you are? To change the way you eat, the activities you do, the places you go, and possibly the people you socialize with? Are you ready to leave the comfort of familiarity and start the difficult process of truly changing the things about you that have made you overweight? Are you ready to give up what you've been using as a crutch for so long?

> *If you think that you can be the exact same person you are*
> *now, just in a thinner body, then you're mistaken.*

Lifestyle change is actually *life change*. You will be a different person if you successfully complete this process. Do you want to be that person? Most importantly, ask yourself whether you are ready to change *now*. Beginning a behavior change effort before you are truly ready greatly increases your odds of failing.[1] Are you ready?

## ✐ Exercise 2: Decide Whether You Want to Make the Effort.

Spend a few minutes journaling about whether you really want to make the effort to change your life. You might use a pros/cons list or just write down the emotions you're feeling about this right now.

To get you started, do this: Close your eyes and imagine your life ten years from now. Imagine that you change nothing. You continue to follow the same eating habits; you make no effort to increase your daily level of activity; you spend the same number of hours every day in a car, at a desk, on the computer, and in front of the TV. Your habits do not change, but your body does. The natural process of aging (left unchecked) is slowing your metabolism, degrading your immune system, and causing what muscles you have now to shrink and atrophy.

What do you look like? How do you move? Do you have trouble getting up from a chair, out of the car, or out of bed in the morning? Are you walking with a limp or a shuffle? What's your breathing like as you walk down the hallway or up a flight of stairs? Are you sick often? Does your back hurt? How many different medications are you taking? What does a typical day look like for you? Are you able to work, to complete errands or other routine tasks, to tend to your family responsibilities? Is there anything physically enjoyable about your life at all?

The future you have just imagined is yours. It is your *inevitable* future if you do nothing to alter it. It's not likely that you've imagined a life worse than what will come to be—when it comes to our health, we tend to be overly optimistic. Diabetes, heart attacks, and strokes happen to "other people," not you. You imagine that you'll carry on just as you are today. And even if the state you're in today is not very good, you're still managing, right? But how much longer will you manage? How long do you have until this imagined future becomes your reality?

The good news, of course, is that you can do something to alter your future. You can start today. It's as simple as making up your mind—just choose to reject that ominous future and transform it into something that is worlds better. This time imagine the future you will have if you start down the path of healthier living. Ask yourself all of those same questions again, but this time imagine that you are thinner and fitter ten years from now.

One of these scenarios will be your reality. Your actions from this point on will manifest the one or the other.

## Character Example

Samantha is a fifty-four-year-old lawyer with a midsized firm. She is five feet five inches tall and weighs 220 pounds. She's been on medication for hypertension and elevated triglycerides for three years. She exercises sporadically and tries to eat as well as she can, but her work schedule doesn't make it easy. She has a history of losing fairly large amounts of weight and then regaining it back over the course of several months. She is married with three teenaged children, and her life is busy and stressful. She is the primary breadwinner in the household and travels two or three times per month for work. In her notebook, Samantha writes:

*Exercise 2: Do I Want to Make This Effort?*

*After closing my eyes and imagining my life ten years from now, I am sad. I don't want to look like this anymore. I don't want to feel this tired, or worry that my clothes won't fit, or see that look on someone's face when I point to the empty seat next to them on the airplane ("Oh, great—I get to sit next to the fat woman!"). I'm scared too, though.*

*I don't know if I can take on a project this big right now, with everything going on at work and at home. The kids' schedules are crazy, my schedule is crazy, and I don't know if I can add one more thing right now. I know I eat badly when I'm stressed. I use food as a comfort when I'm tired or anxious or upset (which is a lot these days). I want to do something about this, but I just don't know if I can do it now. I don't think I can give up the only thing that gives me a little bit of comfort or pleasure in an otherwise frantic life.*

## Character Example

Cindy is twenty-nine years old, single, and works in Human Resources at the local state university. She has been moderately overweight her whole life, but last weekend, she was horrified to read "192.6" when she stepped onto her scale. This is the most weight she has ever carried on her five-foot-eight frame, and the thought of weighing 200 pounds and of still being single at the age of thirty are unbearable to her. She has been a lifelong exerciser, but is also a self-admitted carb-a-holic. Sweets, and especially chocolate, are her downfalls. She often eats out of boredom when she's alone at night. She also frequently goes out with friends or colleagues after work for happy hour, often just because she doesn't want to go home and be alone. In her notebook, Cindy writes:

*Exercise 2: Do I Want to Make This Effort?*

*After imagining the different possibilities for my life ten years from now, I DEFINITELY know that I want to get started on this right away!! I am willing to do whatever it takes to be sure that I am not in worse shape at thirty-nine than I am today.*

*I have been so ashamed of myself lately. I had to buy new clothes—the biggest size ever—last month, and yesterday I had trouble squeezing into even those slacks. This can't go on anymore. I need to change the way I eat, I know. Maybe change up my workout too. I know it's not going to be easy, and I'll have to make some big sacrifices. What I've tried in the past hasn't worked so I need to find a new way. I'm excited about it, though, and ready to get started!*

If, like Samantha, you are unsure or you know you're not ready to try this right now, that's okay! It's better to be crystal clear about what you want, how hard you're willing to work, and how much you're willing to sacrifice for it at the outset. Rather than spending your time and energy going through the motions of a process you're not 100 percent invested in, you can use that time and energy doing things that actually *are* a priority for you right now. And if losing weight continues to hang in the back of your mind, if it's something you keep coming back to, then use this time to educate yourself and prepare for the day when you're ready to take the plunge. You can continue reading this book through to the end for informational purposes and to get a better idea of what will be involved when you *are* ready to change; you can subscribe to a favorite health and fitness magazine; you can try out a new exercise class, take a healthy cooking class, and so on. You can take small steps right now to test the waters and see if, at some point, you will be ready for the really big effort of permanent lifestyle change. *But you need to be realistic about the outcomes of those activities.* Don't expect big changes from small efforts. Use them, instead, as practice for the big dance, or as a way to achieve smaller but potentially important goals, like maintaining your current weight, boosting your mood, gauging your level of motivation to start the program, and so on.

If you're feeling gung-ho and ready to go like Cindy, then congratulations! You're ready to answer the next big question.

## Do You *Believe That You Will* Lose the Weight and Keep It Off?

I am sure that many of you are saying, "I don't know. I've tried so many times before and always wound up back in the same place. I've been overweight for so long, I can't remember what it was like to be thin." And it's perfectly normal and understandable for you to feel that way. Past success or failure is the greatest influencer on present self-confidence. If you have failed in the past, you'll find it hard to believe you can succeed now, but I am telling you that you must! Behavioral research has shown that the belief in your ability to change is one of a few key determinants of your success. Not only that, but a direct circular relationship exists between that belief and your subsequent actions: if you believe that you can change, you will take actions toward your goals, and when you are actively working toward your goals, your confidence in your ability to change increases.[2]

I'm not telling you to forget the past—you'll use your past weight-loss experience as a valuable tool when planning the road ahead. I am, however, telling you to forget your past *failures*. You're a different person now. Your life circumstances are different, you're a little older and a little wiser, you're more committed now than you were before, and you have this new, vital information at your disposal. So change your thinking right now, and believe that *you will be successful*!

Here are two important exercises designed to help you do this:

 ## Exercise 3: Practice Positive Self-Talk.

Your weight isn't something you are proud of, and consequently, you probably have a lot of negative self-talk going on in your head a lot of the time. Right now, on a scratch piece of paper *not* in your notebook, I want you to write down all of the usual negative phrases you think to yourself or even say to others about yourself. Don't limit these phrases to those pertaining only to your weight—it's important for you to identify *all* of your negative thinking here. This should take some time. Think hard and try to cover everything. Write about how you look, how you feel, what you aren't able to do, why you have failed in the past, whether you perceive others to like you or not—everything!

Now, on the next blank page in your notebook, write a sentence or a phrase at the top that will prompt you to think positively about yourself and this process. For example, at the top of the page you might write, "I believe I will succeed," or, "I am strong, capable, and beautiful." Then, below that sentence, transform each one of those negative scratch-paper statements into its positive opposite. For instance, if one of your statements is, "I am never committed enough to keep up a regular exercise program," then your new statement is, "I am committed to keeping up a regular exercise program." Do that for *every* negative statement.

When you've finished, throw away the scratch paper full of negative statements. Read your positive statements five times, right now. Read them every morning when you wake up and every night before you go to bed for the next week. And this week, every time you catch yourself talking or thinking negatively about yourself, replace that statement with its positive opposite, and add it to your notebook. You will quickly learn to notice negative thinking and put a stop to it, and you'll reframe your world as one of positive capability if you faithfully practice this very simple exercise.

## Character Example

On a piece of scratch paper, Bob writes the following negative statements:

- *My athlete days are long, long gone. Now I'm just a big fatty.*
- *I can never stick with a weight-loss program long enough to get the results I want.*
- *Dieting only works for a short time for me.*
- *I hate to exercise!*
- *People judge me, think of me differently (negatively) because I am fat.*
- *My wife is probably going to leave me, and I can't blame her.*
- *My kids think I'm a big loser, and they are right.*
- *The other advisors at the firm are better at their jobs than I am.*
- *People sometimes look at me like I'm some kind of freak.*
- *I can't control my food cravings, especially when I'm out with family or friends.*
- *Sometimes I feel like food is more important to me than anything else.*

Then, in his notebook, Bob writes:

*Exercise 3: Practice Positive Self-Talk.*
- *I will triumph! Here are some things that are true about me:*
- *I am still an athlete at heart. I can get back in shape and look good again.*
- *I will find the right program for me and stick with it. I'm in this for the long haul.*
- *I will change the way I eat and find the right eating plan for me.*
- *Exercise is hard for me right now because I'm so out of shape, but I will start slowly and work every day to get fit, and one day I will love working out as much as I used to in my college days.*

- *People see me as an equal and they respect me.*
- *My wife loves me, and I deserve her love.*
- *My kids love and respect me, and I am a great father and good role model for them.*
- *I am just as talented as anyone at my firm. My clients are lucky to have me as their advisor.*
- *I am content with the way I look.*
- *I am in control of what and how much I eat.*
- *Food is meant to nourish my body and to be enjoyed, but it is not the most important thing in my life.*

Bob lights the scratch piece of paper with the negative statements written on it on fire and enjoys watching it burn in his kitchen sink. He then reads his list of positive statements five times in a row. With each reading, he works hard to internalize the words. By the fifth reading, he is smiling a little. Over the next week, he reads his list each night before he goes to bed and the first thing when he wakes up in the morning. The first couple of days he catches himself doing a lot of negative self-talk. Whenever he does, he quickly jots down what he was thinking or saying. At the end of the day, he pulls out those statements and converts them all to their positive opposites in his notebook. By the end of the first week, Bob is surprised at how he thinks and says negative things about himself much less frequently. He's really starting to view himself as this new person, and he is generally a lot happier than he was just one week ago. He's excited to move on to the next exercise.

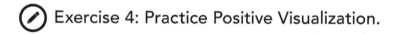 Exercise 4: Practice Positive Visualization.

Visualization is the use of images to create a physical and mental picture of a desired outcome. The more concrete and specific you can make your picture, the better. For example, if you can use actual photos of yourself from a time when you were at your target weight, you'll have a very accurate picture of what you will look like when you reach your goal. If you don't have pictures of yourself, find pictures of people in magazines who represent your future thin, fit self. Of course, you'll have to apply your own "reality filter" when selecting these photos, since the media so often portrays both men and women as overly thin and flawlessly attractive. Cut out pictures of the clothes you will be able to wear and of people doing the activities you will be able to do and tape them into your notebook. If you don't have any magazines on hand, you can create an electronic portfolio using images found online. Then in your notebook create a word picture by describing your body, your clothes, and the kinds of activities your future self will be doing down to the smallest detail. Writing out your word picture is a powerful way to cement it in your mind, and taking it out and reading it often will help you begin to truly visualize your ideal self. What will be most effective in creating that picture is using a combination of physical images, digital images, and a word picture, so don't skip the first part. The more detail you can add to the visualization of your new life, the more effective it will be. This is a very powerful tool because it not only provides you with strong motivation, but it begins to change some of those pathways in the brain.[3] Remember that your mind needs to start seeing you as a fit, thin person, and the best way to do that is to repeatedly expose it to those kinds of images.

## Character Example

Ellen is a forty-eight-year-old police officer, divorced, and the mother of two grown children. She has been slowly but steadily gaining weight since her divorce eight years ago, and is presently in jeopardy of being taken off of patrol duty due to her weight. She is five feet seven and weighs 207 pounds. She needs to lose at least 15 or 20 pounds to keep her patrol beat, but her ultimate goal is to lose 40 or 50 pounds. Ellen digs through a box of photos and pulls out one of her standing next to her daughter at her daughter's high school graduation. Then she digs way into the bottom of the box and pulls out a photo of herself twenty-two years ago, a shiny young police recruit getting her police badge pinned to her uniform. She tapes the photo of her and her daughter up on the bathroom mirror, and she slides the other photo into her work bag. Every morning she looks at herself in the photo next to her daughter and smiles. Throughout the day, she pulls out the photo of her getting her police badge and imagines looking and feeling that capable again.

In her notebook, Ellen writes:

*Exercise 4: Practice Positive Visualization.*

*I'm going to be a fit, strong police officer, worthy of the badge I wear. I'll pass the next physical aptitude test with no trouble at all, and my fellow officers will feel confident in my ability to work with them in any type of situation. On my days off, I'll take Lucky on hikes through the river valley, and I'll join my friends on their long bike rides. My knees and back won't hurt all the time, and I'll be able to plant and tend to a garden again. I'll be the picture of health in my police uniform—and in that chiffon dress I bought in Chicago a few years ago!*

Once you have been practicing positive self-talk and positive visualization for a week or two, you should start to believe that you will achieve your goal. When you feel that happening, it's time to move on and take your first concrete action toward your weight-loss effort. Remember, you're changing mentally so that you can change physically as well.

## Build a Social Foundation for Success

Getting other people involved in your effort may seem odd or even scary, but this exercise is vitally important for two reasons. First, it indicates your frame of mind and your level of confidence in your ability to succeed. Getting others involved in your effort demonstrates to them and to yourself that you are committed, and it adds an important layer of accountability. This can greatly reduce your chance of falling back into your old bad habits.[4]

Your interactions with others can impact your weight-loss effort in another big way: who you spend time with has a big effect on how much you weigh. A 2007 Harvard University study found that the risk of becoming obese increased by 57 percent among people who had one or more close friends who were obese.[5] In a follow-up study, researchers at Arizona State University confirmed the Harvard findings and concluded that the primary reason for this is that we tend to mimic the behaviors of those close to us.[6] So, in this exercise you'll not only involve your social circle in your weight-loss efforts, but you must also determine whether your relationship with them is going to help or hinder your progress.

Many people are gun-shy when it comes to this exercise. Announcing your intentions to others can be scary, especially if you've tried and failed to lose weight in the past. But recognize that this kind of thinking undoes some of the tough work you have just completed—it brings doubt back into your mind, which is the opposite of believing you will lose weight.

*In order to truly believe something, your actions—and not just your thoughts or words—need to reflect that belief.*

By telling others what you are doing, you push outside of your comfort zone and make it more real. Ask yourself: Is part of the reason why you don't want to tell people about your weight-loss effort because you're afraid you might fail? If the answer is yes, then you should go back to Exercises 3 and 4. Getting into the mind-set that success is guaranteed, and that only the rate of progress is in question, is essential. Also, upping your personal stake in the process by making it "public" is a big part of what makes this different from other weight-loss programs.

Your first concrete step toward your weight-loss goal requires that you tell everyone who is important in your life about your weight-loss effort.

When I say "everyone who is important in your life," I really mean everyone with whom you are in regular contact. Your close friends, your spouse or partner, and other family members, but also your boss, your coworkers, and those friends you see on a more occasional basis (monthly or more frequently).

There are different ways you can go about telling the various people in your life about your weight-loss efforts, and the technique you use with each will largely depend on what type of relationship you have with them. For example, it's probably best to sit down in person with immediate family members and your closest friends for a true heart-to-heart talk. Let them see on your face how important this is to you, so that they understand the opportunity they have to help you succeed.

For more casual acquaintances and coworkers, an e-mail or post on social media is probably adequate—it gets the word out to many and makes them aware that you're doing this. But where your boss is concerned, I encourage you to have a face-to-face conversation. Whether your relationship with this person is a good one or a not-so-good one, he or she holds a position of power over you, and therefore it is a very significant relationship, whether you recognize that or not. Talking to your boss in person, letting him or her know that this is a serious endeavor and one that is very important to you, and then *asking for his or her support* can give you an added psychological edge you would not otherwise have. Feeling that you have the support of someone in a position of authority is a huge boost, even if you don't particularly care for that person. And, equally important, your boss may be in a position to offer you other kinds of concrete help, such as access to a workplace gym or reduced rates at the facility of your choice; bringing in healthier food options to the workplace cafeteria or vending machines; or offering healthier food and snack options at company meetings. Some employers are now even offering employer-paid weight-loss counseling services as part of their benefits packages. So don't pass up this opportunity to gain support at the place where you spend at least half of your waking hours!

You may be wondering about the people you "don't like" at work or who "don't like" you. We all have at least one or two of those people in our lives. In most cases it's fine to skip over these people and not bother telling them, but be honest with yourself about why you are choosing to do so. If it's because you truly don't care, then that's okay. But if you're secretly afraid that you will fail and you don't want them to know, then you don't really believe in yourself and you need to go back and do some more work on your earlier exercises.

It's important for you to be prepared for the possibility that as you tell the people in your life about your efforts, you may find one or two of them who are less than excited for you. They may feel threatened by your plans to lose weight because it will affect them in what they see as a negative way. Understand that their reaction is about *them* and not about you. And then ask yourself whether this person will be a help or a hindrance to you. In fact, you should make this distinction for every person on your list. Even those who seem very supportive and happy for you might end up being bad influences. If your usual interactions with them include activities or behaviors you no longer want to participate in, then they may fall in the "detractor" camp. Don't worry too much right now about how to address this—we'll go over some ways to manage these relationship dynamics later, in chapter 12. For now, just start to become aware of who is in your circle of supporters and what that circle looks like.

## 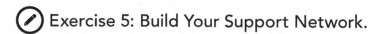 Exercise 5: Build Your Support Network.

Make an extensive list in your notebook of everyone close to you, and place a checkmark by their name as you tell each of them about your endeavor in whatever way you choose. After you see how they respond, divide your list into four categories: Super Supporters,

Supporters, On the Fence, and Detractors. Super Supporters are those handful of family members or friends whom you will turn to time and again for encouragement, guidance, and accountability. Supporters are those who are happy for you and are not likely to put you into tough situations. Those you categorize as On the Fence are friends who will be happy for you, but only if it means you won't change (which, of course, you will). They might be brought around through the use of effective communication and effort on your part. A Detractor is anyone—no matter how close a relationship you have with them— who will continually tempt you to break your new habits or who is openly against your weight-loss effort. They may say things like, "Come on, you can have this just this one time," or "I don't understand why you're doing this anyway—you look fine!"

## Character Example

For Exercise 5, Bob spends more than an hour listing everyone he can think of who plays an important role in his life. After recalling from memory all of the most obvious people—close friends, family, his boss, and coworkers he interacts with regularly—he then scans his e-mail contact lists, his Facebook friends and LinkedIn contacts, and even his high school and college yearbooks. He's surprised at how many people he had forgotten about! He makes himself write down the names of everyone who is important to him, and not just the people he *wants* to share this information with. He tries not to assume who might or might not be supportive or judgmental. Rather, he reminds himself that he should be excited to tell everyone he knows about this, because he *believes* that he will succeed.

At the end of the day, Bob has a list of eighty-seven names. Right away, he contacts about two-thirds of those via e-mail and social media, making a general announcement about his weight-loss efforts and asking for any support he can get. For the remaining twenty or so people, he makes phone calls or appointments to meet in person. His wife and son already know about his intention to lose weight, but that night at the dinner table, he makes it official and tells them what that really means:

"You both know that I'm trying to lose weight again," he begins. "But this time it is going to be different. This time I'm not trying any crash diets or insane exercise programs. I won't be losing a lot of weight in a short amount of time. In fact, by my calculations, it will probably take over two years to get to where I want to be. But I know that I can do it, and if I have your help and support, it will be a lot easier.

"This will mean some changes for all of us. I won't be bringing home fried chicken or ordering pizza for dinner anymore. I might be kind of cranky for the first few weeks once I start trying to change my diet. We'll have to cook more meals at home, which means more grocery shopping. I know that will probably fall to you, honey [referring to his wife], since I get home so late most evenings. But I'll try to shop on the weekends and help cook up some healthy meals too. I want to do it right this time, and I hope we all get a little healthier in the process."

After he has told everyone on his list and gotten a sense of their reactions to his declaration, he puts each person's name under one of the four categories. He's happy to see that he has a solid group of five Super Supporters and another eight people on the Supporter list. There are only three people he's listed as Detractors, but he is surprised at how many of his friends and family seem to be On the Fence. He'll have some work to do later if he is to maintain his friendships with these individuals without compromising his efforts.

## Chapter Two

# DO YOUR RESEARCH

You've already done some great work and laid the foundation for a successful program. Now it's time to turn your attention toward one component of your weight gain—food. Before you can decide what your dietary goals will look like, you need to assess where you're starting. In this important chapter, I ask that you make an honest assessment of your eating habits. I am not asking you to change them—just the opposite, in fact. I'm asking you to do nothing differently during this phase so that you can get the most accurate picture possible. I'd also ask that you not judge what you see, but just observe. Getting down on yourself and wallowing in feelings of shame or guilt will not be a productive use of your mental energy. Remember that you've decided to change your life! Focus on what lies ahead.

## Step Three:

## SEE EXACTLY WHERE YOU'RE STARTING FROM

By learning exactly what your current diet looks like, you'll be able to pinpoint which specific changes you'll need to make in the near future. In order to get an accurate assessment, you'll have to collect some very detailed information about what, when, and how much you eat and drink, and I mean all of it—every bite, nibble, sip, and gulp. Everything you eat and drink will need to be accounted for, and the only way to do this is by using everyone's least favorite weight-loss tool, the food log. There's no way around it—you have to do it. The good news is that you don't have to do it forever. For now, you only have to log what you eat for seven days. Read on to find out why this exercise is mandatory, what you can expect to gain from it, and exactly how to do it.

## Calories

Personally, I hate counting calories, but I still do it because it's such a key element in maintaining my weight. At this stage of the game I don't do it all the time. For at least one week every other month I keep a detailed food log on an app that totals calories and nutritional data for me. It's my way of staying vigilant and identifying potential pitfalls before they become frequent enough to turn into bad habits.

Because weight loss is ultimately about burning more calories than you consume, you're going to have to get familiar with the value of a calorie, both in terms of food and activity. The only way to really do this is by keeping both a food log and an activity journal. Let's talk more about the food log first.

## The Split Personality of the Food Log

Many, many studies have shown that people who consistently track their food and exercise have better success at losing weight and keeping it off than those who do not.[1] And many studies have also shown that almost no one accurately tracks either their calories consumed or their calories burned.[2] In fact, in the case of most web- and app-based programs or calculators, inaccuracy is, unfortunately, very common.

To be fair to these programs and their developers, I'll admit that most of the inaccuracy in calculating calories consumed is your fault and mine. We are terrible at tabulating the number of calories we consume. We shouldn't feel bad, though, because *everyone* is terrible at it. An analysis of multiple studies that had people track calories consumed showed that subjects underreported that number by between 10 and 45 percent, with the average hovering right around 30 percent.[3] For obese individuals, the data is even worse; a 2013 study found that obese women reported 41 percent fewer calories than they actually consumed—that equated to 853 calories per day, the fat equivalent of over 1.5 pounds per week![4]

So why keep a food log at all if it's so hard to accurately count calories? For starters, although your actual numbers are guaranteed to be off at least by a little, a good food log gives you a useful *estimate* of your average weekly calorie consumption. By the end of your first week, you'll know whether you have a little to worry about, or a lot.

A well-kept food log is also extremely useful for identifying which foods are your "worst offenders." As you begin to track your diet for the first time (or for the first time in a while), you'll be amazed at how many calories are in some of the things you thought were "not that bad" or even "healthy." This, in turn, can help you restructure the makeup of your meals. For example, as you realize that even healthy whole grains have about 200 calories per serving, where vegetables have about 35, you'll start piling more of the brightly colored stuff and less of the drab brown and tan stuff onto your plate. As you get deeper into it, you can further benefit from tracking specific nutrients, like protein, fat, saturated fat, fiber, sugars, and sodium. A good food log can give you a snap-shot look at not just the quantity of calories but also the overall quality of your diet.

The food log is also a great tool for thinking through what you're going to have ahead of time if you plan to eat out at a restaurant. If it's a popular restaurant, and if you're using a program with a good database, the restaurant's menu items will likely be listed, so you can choose the best meal before you even get there.

The last way that a food log is useful is probably the most powerful—it holds you accountable and makes your choices better. Those who track their diets report making better food decisions than they otherwise would,[5] even if no one is looking at the food log but them! Knowing that you are going to have to put down in writing that piece of cake or that third glass of wine makes you really think about whether you want to have it or not, and oftentimes you'll decide that you don't.

As you continue working on the important journaling exercises from Step 2, I want you to also start keeping a food log right away. This is the first concrete step toward building your unique weight-loss program. You absolutely need to know what you're up against in terms of your eating and drinking habits. It may be surprising to you. It may be shocking, in fact, to see just how poorly, or how much, you eat.

I hope that it will also be revelatory and give you great insight into exactly why you've gained weight. Maybe you'll find that you consume most of your calories after 6:00 p.m. Maybe you'll be stunned to learn that you drink a quarter or more of your calories every day. You might be lucky enough to identify a few specific foods that you can cut out and easily save a few hundred calories. The truths that food logs illuminate are different for each person. But you will only find out what those truths are if you are absolutely honest and painstakingly thorough in keeping your food log.

Try as best as you can not to alter the way you eat for one full week. Think of this as a science experiment—you are both the subject and the scientist. Be as accurate as possible, and try to make it a "normal" week for you. Simply observe and record everything, and don't judge or feel guilt or be tempted to make yourself look better on paper than you truly are. Spend one week getting the most accurate data you possibly can. Here's how:

## The Anatomy of a Good Food Log

Regardless of whether you find a smartphone app or use the good old pen-and-paper method, there are a few things you must do in order to maximize the effectiveness of your food log. Remember, this is a key diagnostic tool, but it will only be as useful as it is detailed and accurate.

If you have never logged your food before, you'll quickly find that it has the potential to be quite time-consuming! If you're fortunate enough to have a smartphone or other mobile device, you'll find a bevy of apps available that can cut the time you spend while instantly giving you detailed nutritional information on everything you consume. Many apps even allow you to use your phone's camera to scan the barcode on food items and then all you have to do is select how many servings you had. If you don't plan to use a mobile app, you'll find that many apps also have functional websites—if you can access an Internet-connected computer daily, you can still use this time-saving technology.

For years, I tracked my food and exercise in a 3 x 5-inch notebook. It was simple, portable, and I could customize it to track whatever I wanted. It also allowed me to easily make notes about other things that were affecting my diet and exercise choices that day, like sleep (or lack of), time, special-occasion outings, mood, and injuries. (Many of the apps and websites include a comment field with the food diary, and I highly recommend that you use it to jot down notes, making your log a more complete tool.) The only real drawback to the pen-and-paper method is that it's generally more time-consuming because you have to find the nutritional information (calories, grams of carbs, fat, protein, etc.) on your own. You can easily do this by reading the labels on packaged food items, but you'll need a good comprehensive book or a trusted website to find that information for things like bulk grains, fresh fruits and vegetables, and home-cooked meals (which should eventually make up the bulk of your diet). If you are going to use the pen-and-paper method, get a separate small notebook exclusively for that purpose rather than putting your food entries in your weight-loss program notebook.

Once you've decided how you'll track what you consume, it's time to set up your system.

# ✐ Exercise 6: Keep a Detailed Food Log.

*Without modifying your current diet,* track everything you eat and drink for seven consecutive days. The method you use is up to you, but you will need to accurately document the following key pieces of information:

1. Type of food
2. Meal or snack name (Breakfast, Lunch, Dinner, Snack)
3. Portion size
4. Calories
5. Grams of fat and saturated fat (and grams of sugar for extra credit)
6. What time of day you consumed each meal/snack/beverage
7. Method of preparation
8. Your general attitude, emotions, cravings, level of hunger, and other factors for each day (written out in journal format)

Remember that calories are what determine whether you're losing or gaining weight, so it's important that you track them as accurately as possible. If you're using a web-based program or app, you can also easily track grams of sugar and grams of fat, and I suggest you do so. If you're using pen and paper, it's not necessary at this point.

Portion size is probably the area with the biggest potential for inaccuracy. It also happens to be where hidden calories most often sneak their way onto your waistline. You might be eating a pretty healthy meal or snack, but if you eat a large portion of it, you can still unknowingly sabotage your weight-loss efforts.

If you believe, as I do, that anything worth doing is worth doing properly, then you should go out right away and buy a good digital kitchen scale and use *only* that when measuring portion sizes. Why do I recommend this? Because even standard measuring cups can be slightly off, and the nutritional information on the back of packages is *always* listed by weight, with something like "approx. 1/4 cup" tacked on afterward. Here is built-in inaccuracy. For example, eyeballing a level quarter-cup of walnuts can put you off by as many as 50 calories. But weighing out 30 grams of walnuts will give you the exact calorie and nutrition information every time. So right away, get into the habit of weighing out your portions and ingredients.

The time of day and meal/snack categories of your log entries will be helpful in identifying trends. For example, maybe you regularly have a sugary drink midmorning, or maybe you tend to eat or drink a lot of empty calories in the evenings. By noting the time of your meals, snacks, and beverages, you can easily see trends like these after only a few days' worth of data. Once you've identified those trends, it will be easier in the future to be more mindful about them and make better choices.

Method of preparation is very important because it can radically change the calorie content of a type of food. If you put in your food log: "Dinner, 7:30 p.m., 5 oz. chicken breast, 3 oz. potatoes, small salad with lite dressing" that sounds pretty healthy. But obviously there would be a big difference between a meal consisting of battered and fried chicken strips with home fries, and one that included grilled chicken and roasted potatoes. It is essential that you enter the exact method used to prepare your food. If you're eating at a restaurant and not sure what type of oil was used or how much, ask your server, or at the very least err on the side of caution—choose a method of preparation that estimates more calories rather than fewer. Try to give yourself the most accurate picture possible.

After completing this exercise, you'll likely notice some negative trends in your eating habits. You will use what you learn a bit later to decide which of those behaviors you want to target first. Pay close attention to which foods are "calorie dense" and which are "nutrient dense."

Calorie-dense foods have a lot of calories in a relatively small serving and don't deliver many nutrients, or they deliver a lot of only one or two nutrients. Some examples include oils, pasta, bread, cheese, candy, and other processed, sugary, or high-fat foods. Nutrient-dense foods, on the other hand, have relatively few calories for a standard portion size, and they will be packed with more vitamins, minerals, and fiber. Examples include fruits and vegetables, beans and legumes, lean sources of protein, and whole grains.

If you're using an app or program that does the figuring for you, it can be enlightening to analyze the break-down of macronutrients in your diet—what percentage of your calories comes from fat, protein, and carbohydrate. If you're keeping a log by hand, then I recommend leaving this step for later on, so you don't get too overwhelmed with the amount of time you spend on this.

At the end of your scientific week of study, do a thorough review of your food log and pull out these vital summarizations:

1. What is your daily average for calories consumed?
2. How many grams of fat and saturated fat do you consume per day on average?
3. How many of your daily calories come from beverages? What types of beverages?
4. Is there a particular time of day when you tend to consume a lot of calories?
5. Which foods were higher in calories, fat, or sugar than you thought?
6. What events triggered poor eating? (Work or family stress, busy schedule, out with friends, watching TV, etc.)
7. How did your weekend (Friday–Sunday) daily calorie totals compare with weekdays (Monday–Thursday)?
8. What else did you learn?

## Character Example

Cindy is fairly tech-savvy but doesn't want to use her mobile device, so she decides to use a popular food-tracking website to gather information about the food she's eating. She will also carry a small notebook and pen with her so she can jot down anything she consumes while she's away from her computer. She chose this method of tracking because she doesn't want to have to add up calories and calculate grams of fat on her own. This website will do all of that for her, and even give her easy-to-read reports complete with charts and graphs if she wants them.

Because Cindy is using a website (and the same would be true for an app), she needs to be sure to set the parameters to "Maintain Current Weight" or to lose "0 Pounds Per Week," otherwise she may be tempted to alter her food intake to achieve a preset calorie target. Remember, she doesn't want to restrict her dietary intake at this point. Once she has gotten a good look at her current eating habits, she can go in and modify those settings to match her weekly weight-loss goals. Here's a sample day from Cindy's food log, along with the comments from her journal:

| Breakfast | Quantity | Calories | Carbs | Fat | Protein | Sugar | Sat Fat |
|---|---|---|---|---|---|---|---|
| Breakfast Sandwich | 1 sandwich | 410 | 31 | 15 | 16 | 3 | 7 |
| Coffee, brewed from grounds | 2 cups | 5 | 0 | 0 | 1 | 0 | 0 |
| Half & Half (Circle F) | 1 tbsp. | 20 | 1 | 2 | 1 | 1 | 1 |
| Sugar, white granulated | 1 tsp | 15 | 4 | 0 | 0 | 4 | 0 |
| | Totals | 450 | 36 | 17 | 18 | 8 | 8 |
| Lunch | Quantity | Calories | Carbs | Fat | Protein | Sugar | Sat Fat |
| Chicken Caesar Salad (Zulu) | 13 oz. | 530 | 32 | 30 | 38 | 2 | 8 |
| 100% Juice Mango | 1 bottle, 16oz. | 300 | 72 | 0 | 2 | 60 | 0 |
| | Totals | 830 | 104 | 30 | 40 | 62 | 8 |
| Dinner | Quantity | Calories | Carbs | Fat | Protein | Sugar | Sat Fat |
| Veggie Pizza (Grazie Mille) | 2 slices, 113g | 736 | 93 | 27 | 32 | 15 | 8 |
| Red Wine, cabernet or merlot | 5 oz. | 123 | 4 | 0 | 0 | 1 | 0 |
| Dark Chocolate (Coco's) | 3 pieces, 25g | 126 | 15 | 8 | 2 | 12 | 5 |
| | Totals | 985 | 112 | 35 | 34 | 28 | 13 |
| Snacks | Quantity | Calories | Carbs | Fat | Protein | Sugar | Sat Fat |
| Peanut Butter Cookies | 2 cookies | 200 | 10 | 19 | 7 | 21 | 8 |
| Coffee, brewed from grounds | 2 cups | 5 | 0 | 0 | 1 | 0 | 0 |
| Half & Half (Circle F) | 1 tbsp | 20 | 1 | 2 | 1 | 1 | 1 |
| Tortilla Chips (Sun Lake) | 16 chips, 140g | 18 | 7 | 2 | 0 | 1 | |
| Salsa (Pablo Picantes) | 3 tbsp | 15 | 3 | 0 | 0 | 0 | 0 |
| | Totals | 258 | 21 | 23 | 9 | 23 | 9 |
| | | Calories | Carbs | Fat | Protein | Sugar | Sat Fat |
| | Daily Totals | 2,523 | 273 | 105 | 101 | 121 | 38 |

*Wow, I can't believe how many calories are in some of the foods I thought were kind of healthy! That chicken Caesar salad has as many calories as a hamburger. And I thought that by always getting the veggie pizza instead of sausage and pepperoni I was doing myself a big favor.*

*I was hungry after the small lunch and had chips and salsa later. I really wanted a soda too, and I have to admit, if I hadn't been keeping this food log, I probably would have. I know I'm not supposed to change anything, but it's amazing how hard it is not to!*

*Today was a pretty regular day—nothing too stressful or anything like that. I got to bed late last night and was dragging all morning, so I needed the second cup of coffee. Once I had the coffee, I couldn't resist the peanut butter cookies my coworker brought in. They were so good!*

*This is a real eye-opener. Look at all those grams of sugar and saturated fat!*

At the end of the week, Cindy looks over her food log carefully and has the website generate reports on calories, fat, saturated fat, and sugar. Then she answers the key questions about her current eating habits:

1. *Average Daily Calories: 2,787*
2. *Percentage of Calories from Fat: 35 percent; Saturated Fat: 16 percent*
3. *Average Daily Calories from Beverages: 450 (wine, coffee drinks, juice)*
4. *It looks like I consume a lot of calories all day long! I did notice that on days when I was stressed at work I snacked after work and drank more wine with dinner.*
5. *Almost everything I usually eat surprised me. That supposedly healthy juice has 60 grams of sugar! It seems like salads are loaded with fat and calories. Pizza, pasta, and Mexican food are all off the charts—even if I try to choose the healthier versions or leave out the guacamole, sour cream, etc. I honestly don't know what I'm going to be able to eat.*
6. *Work stress made me eat and drink more in the evening. Anytime a coworker brought in treats, I couldn't resist them.*
7. *The weekend was only a little worse than weekdays. I went out for happy hour on Friday and that was a calorie disaster, but not as bad as Sunday's brunch out with my sister—I had no idea how bad eggs Benedict were!*
8. *I eat a lot of fat and a lot of sugar. More than 10 percent of my calories come from drinks. I think it will be fairly easy to cut back there. As for the rest of it, I didn't think I was eating that* badly, *but I am going to really have to make some changes. I'm not looking forward to it.*

After you've done your own food log exercise for one week, tuck this information away. You'll use it later, when it's time to identify which dietary behaviors you want to work on first. If there are one or two obvious things you think might be easy to improve right away, then go ahead and take action on them. But don't get too wrapped up in making changes just yet. First, we need to address the important task of goal setting.

# Chapter Three

# WHAT, WHY, AND HOW

**N**ow you have a good idea of where you're starting from, and you're probably getting a sense of how big an undertaking this will be. Before you jump right in and start worrying about exercising more or eating less, I want you to expand your focus, zoom out, and take a look at the big picture again.

By setting up a logical framework for your weight-loss program, you greatly increase your chances for success. In this chapter you will define exactly what you will do, you'll tell yourself why you are doing it, and you'll learn about one of the biggest traps you should avoid.

## Step 4:
## DEFINE YOUR GOALS

### Say Exactly What You Will Do

You've decided that you want to lose weight and you believe that you will do it. You've tracked your food and beverages to see what you're up against, so now it's time to set some goals. This step is crucial because you will need to determine exactly what "losing weight" really means for you.

In weight loss, as in other pursuits, the simple mistake of not setting a good goal at the beginning can spell failure. The two most common mistakes in goal setting are setting a goal that's not specific enough, or setting a goal that is unrealistic. In the case of a goal that is too vague, success is impossible to define. Good goals define exactly which parameters you will measure, and they set time-bound targets for making progress toward those parameters along the way. When you set your sights too high, though, and make a goal that's unrealistic, success is impossible to achieve. This is a grave mistake—the last thing you want to do is create a situation that sets you up to fail. Your confidence will be destroyed, and you'll give up on the whole effort. So, in order to set yourself up for success, you'll need to define your goals specifically and realistically.

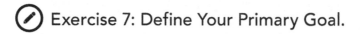

## Exercise 7: Define Your Primary Goal.

Go back in your notebook and read your word picture, look at the pictures you've cut out, or think back to a time when you looked and felt your best. From that image, determine your primary goal. Decide what your specific goal is in terms of pounds or inches lost, clothes size, etc. This is the end result—you in one, three, or five years from now. Now ask yourself, is this realistic? If you are forty years older than the last time you were at your ideal weight, reaching that number again may be unrealistic. Certainly, regardless of how much weight you lose, you'll never look the same as you did back then, because the years take a physical toll on everyone, thin or fat, fit or unfit. So have an honest moment with yourself here and choose a weight or a clothes size or a mental image of your new ideal self that is both desirable *and* attainable. Write that down, as specifically as possible, in your notebook.

Next, you need to figure out how long it's going to take you to transform yourself into that new person. Here is where you must be realistic. Regardless of what certain diets promise or which numbers are available for you to plug into your food log program, the reality is that over the long term, three-fourths of a pound of fat loss per week is the best you should expect. There are individuals who may lose weight more quickly than that, and that's wonderful, but they represent the exception rather than the norm. The general guidance put forth by public health organizations recommends aiming to lose one to two pounds per week,[1] but it's important to note that this recommendation is based on a total weight-loss goal of just 5 to 10 percent of body weight. If you have more than 25 pounds to lose, your rate of weight loss will almost certainly slow as time goes on,[2] so that's why I recommend that you use three-fourths of a pound per week as a best-case scenario for your planning purposes.

Honestly, in my experience, one to two pounds per *month*, or one-fourth to half a pound per week, is more realistic if your weight-loss effort will last longer than eight months. You will likely lose more than this in the beginning, but don't get discouraged when, a few months into your effort, the numbers on the scale begin to eek downward ever more slowly. There are things you can do, which I'll tell you about later, to ensure that your progress doesn't stop altogether, but please take the long view here and set a timeline that accounts for these biological facts. I recommend that you take the number of pounds you came up with in the first part of the exercise above and divide that by one-half to three-quarters a pound. The result will be the approximate number of weeks it should take for you to reach your ultimate goal.

## Character Example

Bob reads his visualization word picture and looks at the photos he collected in Exercise 4. He remembers very well that he wore size 34 jeans in college. While he'd love to get back to that, he wants to be realistic, so he thinks about what weight and clothes size would make him truly happy. He writes the following entry in his notebook:

*Exercise 7: Define Your Primary Goal.*

*I want to lose 130 pounds so that I weigh around 225 pounds; that's about 10 pounds more than I weighed in college. I know I won't look exactly like I did back then—there will probably be a little less muscle and a little more fat—but I'm okay with that. I'd love to fit into size 36 pants again. I may actually have some from way back then!*

Bob gets out his calculator and enters 130/.75. The result is 173.3. This is the estimated number of weeks it will take Bob to lose all of his weight.

*I guess if I'm going to do this right, it's going to take a long time . . . around three years, in fact! That sounds like such a long time, but I have to remember that this is* permanent, *so I might as well just take it one day at a time.*

# Short-Term Goals

Because it's hard to stay focused on the same goal for more than a year, and one of the keys to permanent weight loss is staying focused and motivated the entire time, you need to break down your primary goal into smaller, secondary goals if you have more than 25 pounds to lose. The next exercise is designed to help you do that.

To get started, choose a time frame that your first short-term goal will be bound by. I recommend something longer than one month but not more than six months. In the first month, your body will basically be rebelling against the new changes you're putting it through, so you probably won't see much weight loss. It takes time to unstick your metabolism, and it can be disappointing to set a goal at the one-month mark and find that you seemingly haven't made much progress toward it. Trust me, the progress will come.

In the first month, you should really be focusing on *changing habits*, and not on the result of those changes. By the end of two months, you should start seeing some progress, and it's a good idea to check in occasionally to see if you're on the right track. However, I recommend that you wait to do your first real evaluation at the three- or four-month mark. If you've diligently followed your program for that long and the weight is still coming off more slowly than you'd like, you will know that it's time to make an adjustment. I'll talk about how you can do that in chapter 7.

Again, I recommend you use one-half to three-quarters of a pound per week as a realistic amount of weight you can expect to lose. That's about two to three pounds per month, on average. Don't be tempted to set your goal much higher than this, for *wanting* to lose weight more quickly will not make it so, and failing to meet your unrealistic goals early on can kill your entire weight-loss effort.

Once you have your criteria set, create a new, temporary visual image of yourself—imagine what you'll look like at the end of your time limit. If your initial goal is to lose 10 pounds in three months, visualize what 10 pounds of fat looks like (imagine a large roast, or several small ones). Then imagine those 10 pounds gone from your body. It would be nice if you could pick and choose where the weight comes off first, but it generally comes off a little bit here and a little bit there. You can imagine an inch or two of fat gone from your waistline. Of course, you'll find your arms, hips, neck, and face have all slimmed down too. You might be fitting into a smaller pant size. Take a few moments and get a good mental picture of that in your head. You should also imagine what *feeling* 10 pounds lighter will be like. How much easier will you breathe when walking up a flight of stairs? What kinds of activities will you do with your family that you avoid now? Will you finally be able to touch your toes? See your toes, at least?

## ✎ Exercise 8: Set Your First Interim Goal.

It's time to be specific about the kind of goals you want to set. Weigh the pros and cons of choosing a shorter timeline versus a longer one. Think about your own personality. Are you more apt to be impatient if you pick a longer timeline? How devastating will it be to your effort if you choose a short timeline and don't meet your goal? Most importantly, remember not to set a goal that is overly ambitious. Be honest with yourself about what level of progress will make you happy. Is this really attainable? If not, you'll need to spend some time working on letting go of unrealistic expectations. Keep in mind that you're doing this for the rest of your life—this is a lifestyle change. Short-term diets don't work, only permanent changes do, so take your time and do it right!

## Character Example

Let's see what Bob did with this exercise.

*Exercise 8: Set Your First Interim Goal.*

*I think for my first interim goal, I'll go with Doc's recommendation of losing 35 to 40 pounds in six months. That breaks down to about 1 to 1.5 pounds per week. It's a tall order, but I think I can do it. That will put me at around 325 pounds on August 18.*

*Let me imagine what that will look like: I'll be down two or three inches around my waist, and probably two pants sizes. I have some clothes from when I was that size, so I shouldn't have to buy new. I might be able to see a little muscle definition in my arms—I've always had great guns! It will still be hard for me to climb those stairs at work, but I'll do it, no matter how long it takes or how many times I have to stop to catch my breath. Dragging 40 fewer pounds around should make it easier to get in and out of the car, and I hope to be sleeping a little better at night—if not the apnea, then hopefully at least my back won't ache as much.*

For many people, Bob's initial weight-loss goal of one to one and a half pounds per week might be unrealistic, but because he has a very large amount of weight to lose, he is male, and he has a more muscular body type, this is not an unattainable goal for him. It's important, however, that Bob doesn't stick with this "formula" for subsequent interim goals. As he loses more and more weight, he'll be burning fewer calories given the same activity level (I'll talk more about this later, in part 2). Bob acknowledges this upfront and vows to set realistic interim goals every three to six months, based on how he's progressing. This is definitely a more effective strategy than trying to devise a weight-loss "schedule" that spans three or four years at the outset. If you have a great deal of weight to lose, I recommend that you follow Bob's lead. If you have around 50 pounds or less to lose, however, it can be helpful to break your primary goal down into planned interim time segments right away. It's your choice—just remember that flexibility and adaptability are key to any long-term process. Don't get bogged down in the numbers, regardless of how much weight you ultimately want to lose.

# Step Five:
# DETERMINE *WHY* YOU WANT TO LOSE WEIGHT

## Know What It's All For

Apart from identifying your goals, the next most important factor in this whole process is defining your motivation for achieving them. No matter how motivated you think you are, if your underlying reasons for wanting to lose weight are not important to *you*, you're going to have a hard time sticking with this process over the long term.[3]

Here are some common reasons a person may want to lose weight:

- To reduce health-risk factors (often spurred on by a recent diagnosis of a lifestyle-related disease or precondition)
- To improve self-image and self-confidence
- To attract a mate
- To better one's professional image and/or chances for promotion or career progression
- To improve functional movement and maintain independence
- To make a spouse or partner happy
- To increase energy levels and improve overall mood

- To be able to "keep up with" friends or family members
- To set a good example for children or other family members
- To be able to resume participation in or improve performance of a favorite sport, hobby or other activity

 Exercise 9: List and Categorize Your Motivators.

Make a list in your notebook of all of the reasons why you want to lose weight. There might be many, or only one, and some of your reasons may be different from the examples I've listed above. The important thing is to be honest and tell yourself why you're going through all of this trouble in the first place.

Once you have your list, you need to identify whether each reason is *intrinsic* or *extrinsic*. Intrinsic motivation comes from within you and is linked to positive self-image, enjoyment, or personal satisfaction. Extrinsic motivation comes from outside sources, such as material or social rewards and how other people view you.

Distinguishing between the two can be difficult, so I'll use the list of motivators above and identify them as either intrinsic or extrinsic. Reading each motivator, I am asking, "Is this about the way I perceive myself or the way others perceive me?" Here is how the example list breaks down:

| Intrinsic Motivators | Extrinsic Motivators |
|---|---|
| Reduce health-risk factors* | Attract a mate |
| Improve self-image and self-confidence | Improve professional image and chances for promotion |
| Improve functional movement and maintain independence | Make spouse, partner, or others happy |
| Increase energy levels and improve mood | Keep up with friends and family members |
| Improve performance at a favorite sport/hobby/activity | Set a good example for children or other family members |

\* "Reduce health-risk factors" could be considered extrinsic if your doctor, spouse, or other family member is more concerned about your health than you are.

Now go back to your list and write an *E* next to the goals that are extrinsically motivated, and an *I* next to those that are intrinsically motivated. If your list is comprised of mostly or all *E*s, then you're probably thinking, "Uh-oh, I'm doing this for the wrong reasons!" If all your motivators are extrinsic, then this *is* a problem, but not an insurmountable one. You don't need to give up on your weight-loss goals; you just need to *reframe* your reasons for wanting to lose weight so that this becomes a process that is about *you*. Honestly, if you think about it, virtually everyone who loses weight will realize nearly *all* of the benefits listed above. So, for now, you should reprioritize which of those benefits matter most to *you*.

If your original thought was, "I want to lose weight and get in better shape so I can keep up with my wife on our hiking trip this fall," that motivator will remain valid, of course, but you should tell yourself that your efforts will also result in reduced health-risk factors, improved appearance, higher levels of self-confidence, and you may even decide to start playing tennis again—something you once loved doing, but haven't been able to do in years.

Maybe your spouse has been politely suggesting for months that you try this diet or that exercise class because he or she is worried about your long-term health. Finally, you cave in and agree that you'll try to lose some weight to make your spouse happy. This would be a clear extrinsic motivator, and your chances of succeeding will be pretty slim. If you have come to the decision that you're going to give this weight-loss effort a serious try, then you need to shift your thinking and focus on what *you* are going to get out of this deal. After all, you're the one who will be working and sacrificing. It needs to be important enough to you, or you're likely to give up at the first sign of adversity.

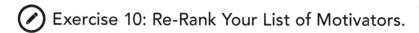 ## Exercise 10: Re-Rank Your List of Motivators.

Look at your list again. Have you thought of any new reasons for wanting to lose weight? Do some of those external motivators seem less important to you now? Go through your positive self-talk and visualization exercises again. Revisit those positive statements and your word picture, and see how they tie into and support your intrinsic motivating factors. Imagine the new you. How do you look? How do you feel? Do you have more energy? How will you use that new energy? What activities might be possible now that weren't before? Are you likely to enjoy physical activities that you didn't used to? Will you spend more time outside? Will your posture or your mannerisms change? How will you present yourself to the world?

Now rank your list of motivators, with the top item being what is most important to you and the bottom one being what is least important. Be honest here—simply writing a list won't do you any good if you aren't backing it up with belief. If you find that extrinsic motivators are still at the top of your list, then you'll need to figure out why you care more about pleasing others than you do about yourself. If you've found that you aren't motivated by any of the intrinsic factors, then it's possible that a lot of your happiness is tied to one or more unhealthy habits, or perhaps you place less value on yourself than you do on others. These are both common scenarios for many people. The key is to work your way out of this kind of thinking—to begin placing the proper value on your health and happiness. Group or individual therapy can be instrumental in helping you find and embrace this value in yourself. You decided in Steps 1–3 that you want to lose weight, believe that you will, and have defined what that means to you, but you can't move forward until you are able to make this process about *you*. You are an important person, and you deserve to live a happy, healthy life!

Once you can say that you're doing this for reasons that are important to you, write down your top two or three motivators on the back of a few business cards. Put one in your wallet, in front of your credit cards, so that you'll see it often, and put the others in places you normally pass by (e.g., the bathroom mirror, the refrigerator, your work desk, etc.). Frequent reminders of why you are losing weight can help you stay on track when you might otherwise succumb to setbacks.

## Character Example

Ellen gets out her notebook and lists all of the reasons why she wants to lose weight:

*Exercise 9: List and Categorize Your Motivators.*
- *I have to lose weight if I want to stay on patrol. I don't want to drive a desk!*
- *If I don't lose weight, it could start seriously affecting my health.*
- *I want to look better in my clothes.*
- *I want to start dating again, and hopefully meet the man of my dreams.*
- *I want to be able to hike like I used to and keep up with my friends on those long bike rides.*
- *I want to feel more confident in my abilities to do my job well. There is a huge physical component to it, and I put myself and the public at risk by being so out of shape.*
- *I want to have more self-confidence and not think that people are always judging me.*
- *I want to be a good role model for my kids.*

Next Ellen goes back to the list and classifies each motivator as either Intrinsic (I) or Extrinsic (E):

- *I have to lose weight if I want to stay on patrol. I don't want to ride a desk! (I)*
- *If I don't lose weight, it could start seriously affecting my health. (I)*
- *I want to look better in my clothes. (I, E)*
- *I want to start dating again, and hopefully meet the man of my dreams. (E)*
- *I want to be able to hike like I used to and keep up with my friends on those long bike rides. (I, E)*
- *I want to feel more confident in my abilities to do my job well. There is a huge physical component to it, and I put myself and the public at risk by being so out of shape. (I, E)*
- *I want to have more self-confidence and not think that people are always judging me. (E)*
- *I want to be a good role model for my kids. (E)*

Next Ellen reorders her list of motivators from most important to least important. As she does so, she also edits each one so that it becomes a powerful motivational statement, rather than just a description:

*Exercise 10: Re-Rank Your List of Motivators*

1. *I will keep my job as a patrol officer.*
2. *I will be able to do my job well and safely.*
3. *I will get healthy and stay that way.*
4. *I will be able to wear whatever I want and look great in it.*
5. *I will start dating again and find the right person for me.*
6. *I will be energetic on hikes with my dog and bike rides with friends.*
7. *I will be a positive role model for my kids; they will be proud of me.*
8. *I won't worry anymore that others are judging me.*

Ellen pins her list of motivators up on her refrigerator door and makes cards with her top three written on the back. She keeps one of them taped to the inside lid of her metal clipboard, where she sees it every time she writes a report or issues someone a ticket. She reads over her list whenever she feels her motivation starting to slip, and before going into tempting, high-risk situations. She uses the list to stay focused on her weight-loss goal and not let her attention be diverted by potential obstacles.

# Step Six:
# DETERMINE WHAT HAS CAUSED THE PROBLEM

## Take Ownership of Your Situation

In the introduction, I told you that your genetic makeup may have been a contributor to your weight up to this point. I also told you about the groundbreaking new science that's proving you can exert control over those genes and make them work for you rather than against you. But for a moment, I'd like you to think about all of the other factors that have led to the condition your body is in—namely, your behaviors. It is my belief—without ever having met you—that your behaviors have influenced your weight more than your genes. On top of that, I'm asserting here that it is possible, *and in fact easy*, for most people to modify their behaviors and overcome those genetic factors, if they only learn how. Here is the proof that has led me to this conclusion:

Over the past seven years, I've worked with dozens of clients who have wanted to lose significant amounts of weight. Many of them have been very successful, and a few of them never lost a pound. At first I was willing to blame genetics—some people's bodies just wanted to hold on to fat more than others. But after changing my training techniques a couple of years ago, I started seeing unmistakable trends that differentiated the successes from the failures. I started gathering much more written and verbal data from my clients about their weight histories, their current attitudes toward weight loss, and their level of confidence in their ability to lose weight, and I found that the way clients answered these questions had everything to do with their success rates.

Without exception, everyone said they had tried many times to lose weight over the years. About 80 percent of them reported that at some point in the past they had lost a significant amount of weight, only to gain it back. When I asked them how they had lost the weight, they reported the usual methods—food tracking, healthier eating, dietary support groups or weight-loss books, increased activity, etc. When I asked them what was going on in their lives at that time, they reported that things were going pretty well. Many of them were gearing up for a big event (weddings, vacations, reunions, etc.), and they were highly motivated to lose the weight. And when I asked them why they thought they gained the weight back, they told me they had gotten off-track and given up their diet and exercise regimens. Upon further questioning, they often reported one of two scenarios: either the big event they'd been preparing for had come and

41

gone so their source of motivation had disappeared, or there had been a major life event (often negative) that intervened and took priority over their new healthy lifestyle.

All of this made perfect sense to me and to them. It was easy to see both how they had been successful and what had happened to return them to their former, unsuccessful habits—and *it had nothing to do with biology or genetics.* The argument that "I just can't lose weight," which many of them came through my door with, was proven false by their own testimonies. They did, in fact, have great success at losing weight, but then the formula they were following changed, and the weight loss stopped. The reason why they were overweight was universally the same: they took in more calories than they burned on an ongoing basis. Of course, they each had very different individual *underlying reasons* for this, but none of those reasons had to do with their genetic predisposition to become fat. They had taken a temporary view of their new healthy habits, had chosen new habits that were unsustainable, or both. As for the 20 percent who had never successfully lost weight in the first place, they simply hadn't used sound methods. They either relied on fad diets that couldn't be sustained or tried exercising (often sporadically) without paying any mind to diet and calorie consumption.

The key to lasting weight-loss success, then, is finding a set of effective habits that you can maintain for a lifetime. In order to do that, I'd like you to start by taking a good look at what *hasn't* worked for you up to now.

It's the nature of our modern society to place many things higher on the priority list than our own health. This is a huge reason why many people today are so unhealthy. Figuring out how you're going to reverse that trend starts with learning to make your health a top priority, and acknowledging that

*Your everyday actions will define either*
*your success or your failure.*

This means taking ownership of the entire weight-loss process and learning that you must choose to take the right actions time after time. Your genetic makeup can make your process take longer than you'd like, but it is not powerful enough to stop you altogether. Thinking that factors other than your behaviors (such as genetics or outside influences) have caused your weight gain is a trap you must avoid. It's time to come clean.

# ✎ Exercise 11: Tell Yourself Why You Are Overweight.

This is a hard exercise for everyone. Many people, in fact, will only perform a shallow, cursory review of the factors that have led to their current condition, without digging deep enough to discover the true cause. Don't let yourself fall into this camp. This exercise requires deep digging, soul searching, and self-honesty. You need to say to yourself, "I am responsible for the condition that I'm in," and then list all of the behaviors that have contributed to that over the years.

> In your notebook, in list or journal format, write down exactly why you are overweight. Do you binge-eat late at night? Do you stress-eat when other areas of your life feel out of control? Do you eat out of boredom? Are you addicted to alcohol, sugar, chocolate, pizza? Is eating the only thing that really makes you happy? Do most of your calories come from beer, wine, or cocktails? Do you eat huge amounts of food when you're out with friends? It's impossible for me to write every potential contributing factor here, but I'm sure that you know your own factors very well, whether you'd like to admit to them or not.

Watch out for the tendency to blame outside influencers: other people, a lack of time, a dislike of healthy foods, or a lack of cooking know-how. Rather, admit to yourself that all of these things are actually in your control: you choose how to spend your time, what kinds of foods you eat, whether to cook your own meals or go out, and whether to devote time to learning how to prepare healthier meals. Again, these are just a few examples, and you must come up with your own list of behaviors. Be exhaustive—leaving things out will just guarantee that they will pop up and get in your way later on.

Now look at what you've written and know that it is the truth, but don't let yourself feel guilty or ashamed about it! While ownership is essential to this process, guilt and self-blame are obstacles that will hinder your progress. Take a rational view of your past behaviors—know them well, because they are the enemy, but know also that you can learn how to bring them under your control and change them permanently.

## Exercise 12: Figure Out Why those Behaviors Exist.

Now that you know which behaviors have made you overweight and you've taken owner-ship of them, it's time to make a list of all of the causal factors that trigger those behaviors.

First, let's define *causal factors*. Causal factors are the prompts or signals that tend to cause you to take a certain action. They can be thought of as the many reasons why you end up eating too much or exercising too little. They can be big things or small, and they can come from your external environment or from within you. Using the example of habitual sleep deprivation as a negative behavior, some causal factors might include being overly stressed, not effectively planning your time, eating or drinking alcohol too late at night, spending time on the computer right before bedtime, or letting the dog sleep on the bed. You can see how specific you will need to get for each of the behaviors you listed above. Don't rush through this exercise. Take your time and list *every single thing* that contributes to your weight-gain behaviors day in and day out.

You should come back to this exercise often as you go through subsequent steps and discover more things that are standing in your way. Seek to identify the small but significant details. Maybe you wrote down in Exercise 11 that you are prone to eating a lot when you go out with friends. In this exercise you break it down: Do you *always* overeat when you're out with friends, or only with certain friends, or only at certain restaurants? Maybe you recognized that you eat the bulk of your calories late in the evening. Here is the chance to figure out why. Are you bored? Have you not eaten frequently enough throughout the day? Or is it just a mindless habit borne of association (I *always* eat popcorn when I watch a movie, for example)? To get a better idea of how thorough and specific you should be, take a look at the character example for Exercises 11 and 12.

## Character Example

Cindy takes a moment to review her seven-day food log, then turns to the next blank page in her journal and writes the following:

*Exercise 11: Tell Yourself Why You Are Overweight.*

*I'm overweight because I have let myself go. I don't make time to exercise, and I don't pay enough attention to my diet. I'm easily persuaded by my friends to skip workouts and eat out (where I almost always make poor food choices and have too many drinks). When I have tried to diet and exercise, I've taken a drastic approach and thought of it only as a temporary effort. I always give up soon after I start. The specific behaviors that have caused me to gain all of this weight are:*

- *I don't exercise regularly at all.*
- *I sit at a desk all day long and make no effort to get up and move around, unless it's to go get a snack or a fattening coffee drink.*
- *I had no idea, up until last week's food log exercise, what I was really eating and what that meant in terms of calories. Even many of the things I thought were healthy actually had a ton of calories.*
- *I go out with friends way too often, and I exercise poor judgement when I do. I eat whatever everyone else wants from the appetizer list and frequently have two or three glasses of wine.*
- *I eat anything and everything that my coworkers bring into work. I am guilty of bringing in these fattening "treats" pretty often too.*
- *I have a large, sweetened coffee drink several days per week. Now I know that one of those drinks has over 300 calories all by itself—never mind the cookie, brownie, or muffin I usually have with it!*

*Exercise 12: Figure Out Why those Behaviors Exist*

*The specific things that cause these behaviors are:*

- *I don't exercise regularly at all.*

  *I mismanage my time and never work it into my schedule. I haven't made it a priority.*

  *I make tons of excuses: I blame the weather, lack of sleep, a busy schedule, whatever.*

  *Honestly, I don't enjoy exercise, so I avoid it.*

  *I have let my gym membership lapse (because I wasn't using it, so I considered it a waste of money), and I don't have any equipment at home.*

- *I sit at a desk all day long and make no effort to get up and move.*

  *I am just lazy; it's easy for me to sit all day.*

*I don't think about getting up unless there's some reason to.*

*It's cold in the hallways and bathrooms, so I try to stay in my office.*

• *I don't pay attention to what I eat.*

*I do this on purpose. I know a lot of the things I eat are bad for me, but they make me feel good, so I just don't think about the calories.*

*I mindlessly eat whenever I watch TV at home.*

*I am a slave to the power of suggestion. If I see someone eating or drinking something on TV, I often get up and mine the refrigerator or pantry.*

*I also stress-eat a lot, at work when I'm up against a deadline or in social situations where I'm uncomfortable (including at extended family gatherings). These social situations often result in consuming alcohol too.*

*I haven't taken the time or made the effort to educate myself about what I'm eating. It didn't take that much work to learn that the salads and juice drinks I thought were healthy were actually calorie disasters!*

• *I eat out often and make poor choices.*

*I know I do this out of fear of being alone. I find going home to an empty apartment depressing.*

*I really do enjoy spending time with my friends. I wish they had healthier habits of their own. I don't want to stop hanging out with them.*

*Again, I have difficulty saying no to something when I see or smell it. I don't know if I can go out and eat something healthy while everyone around me is eating the kind of food I love.*

• *I frequently eat baked goods and other junk food at work.*

*Boredom is one reason for this.*

*Again, seeing and smelling these treats makes it almost impossible for me to resist them.*

*Even if I've been able to resist the food on my own, I always give in when someone offers it to me.*

*I feel like I might offend whoever brought the food in if I don't take any.*

• *I drink a large, sweetened coffee drink several times per week.*

*Again, this is partially out of boredom. It's a reason for me to leave my desk.*

*I often go get the coffee at the invitation of a coworker. It's hard for me to say no to others.*

*I've come to think of this as a reward for work, especially when I've just completed something especially demanding or unpleasant. I've noticed that lately I look for any reason to reward myself, and these trips to the café happen more frequently.*

You might have a longer list of behaviors than Cindy does, or maybe there really are only a few bad habits that have caused your weight gain. The important thing is to know what they are, and to think about every possible influence that causes them. Note that in her statements, Cindy took ownership for all of her behaviors and their causal factors. She did not, for example, say, "My coworkers bring in fattening food all the time," or "My friends drag me out to happy hour two nights a week." It is crucial that you make the same kinds of distinctions. It is easy to blame other people or circumstances for our behaviors, but the truth is that we each ultimately have control over our own actions.

## Is Your Metabolism Dead?

At this point, I want to bring up an issue that may apply to some of you. If you've just gone through the last two exercises and are scratching your head, thinking, *But I don't overeat. I track my calories religiously and eat a healthy diet. I exercise five days a week for an hour each day. I've been doing this for months now, and I can't lose a pound!* I'd like to discuss one possible reason for this.

If you are really honest with yourself, and you do exercise a lot and you have been eating healthy and tracking your calories, then it's possible that your metabolism is so damaged that your body is just in survival mode, hoarding whatever fat and calories you're giving it. The primary reason why this happens is too much dieting. If you're a lifelong dieter who has been yo-yoing in weight for years, or if you've been strictly following a low- or very low-calorie diet (such as a liquid meal replacement or mainstream fad diet), then your body probably thinks it is starving.

Early on, you may have lost a large amount of weight on one of these diets, but the long-term problem with them is twofold: First, they simply don't give your body enough of what it needs to maintain a healthy metabolism, so the body compensates by lowering your metabolism to its bare minimum. Second, the incredibly restrictive nature of these diets makes them impossible to maintain, and when you return to eating a higher number of calories, you're feeding them to a body that has learned to live on less. The result is rapid weight regain, frequently beyond whatever you had lost.

I've worked with several clients who were in this situation. They were habitual dieters, some of whose eating behaviors could be classified as disordered. They had been active their entire lives (often gymnasts or dancers), only to find that as they grew older, they could no longer lose or even maintain weight no matter how drastically they cut their calorie intake. My advice to these clients? *Eat more.* They would have to slowly build their metabolism back up to normal levels through months of careful meal planning and smart exercise programming. Their bodies would have to learn how to run at full capacity again. This was a very slow and methodical process, and not one that you can be guided through in the pages of a book.

If you routinely eat 1,200 or fewer calories per day, exercise regularly, feel severely fatigued and sluggish, have a low immune system, and have been unable to lose weight, then you have a compromised metabolism. It's possible that the cause of that compromise could be hormonal, so I first recommend that you see your physician and/or an endocrinologist to rule out the possibility of a thyroid disorder or other possible medical causes. If nothing is found in your tests, then it's likely you've been slowly sabotaging your metabolism over months or years. Then you'll need to seek out a qualified dietitian or health coach to help get you back on track.

## Chapter Four

# TIME TO TALK ABOUT FOOD

It's time to zoom back in now and take a look at the concrete things that have really contributed to your weight gain: food and lack of, or incorrect, exercise. In this chapter and the next, I'll give you some key information to help you choose from among the many different diet and exercise options available to you, and guide you through the first steps in implementing behavior change in those areas. So, for a moment, set aside your long list of behaviors and causal factors from Exercises 11 and 12, and let's focus on the bigger picture where diet is concerned.

## Step Seven:
## START WATCHING WHAT YOU EAT

### Diet Is a Four-Letter Word, Sometimes

If you've ever tried to lose weight, you have most likely "gone on a diet." In that sense, the word *diet* refers to an eating scheme that severely limits calories, types of food, or entire macronutrient categories (fat, protein, or carbs). These diets can bring quick success, but unfortunately that success usually evaporates just as quickly as it came, often resulting in further weight gain.[1] Once you realize that the diet is impossible to stick with and you return to your pre-diet eating habits, the weight comes back quickly, and many times you can end up a pound or two *heavier* than when you started. This version of "diet" is a four-letter word that you should permanently strike from your vocabulary.

However, if you've used a sound weight-loss program in the past, then you know the term *diet* actually refers to a sustained pattern of eating habits. If you followed a healthy diet for a good length of time, you probably found that you lost weight more slowly but consistently, kept if off for a longer period of time, and only started to regain the weight after you reverted to your old, less-healthy habits.

From this moment on, for the rest of your life, you are to think of "diet" by this second definition, and never, ever be tempted to "go on a diet" again, no matter how trendy it sounds or how fantastic the infomercial models selling it might look. (I can assure you, they did not get those bodies simply by following that diet, and I would be skeptical as to whether they have actually even tried the diet themselves.)

Your systematic approach to losing weight and keeping it off requires that you follow a specific way of eating. Happily for you, I am not going to tell you what that diet should be. How could I possibly know which way of eating is best for you when I've never even met you? I don't know your likes and dislikes, your food allergies or intolerances, or your ethnicity. I have no idea whether you've been diagnosed with hypertension and need to be on a low-sodium diet, or have a high risk for heart disease and need to limit saturated fat. What I do know, and what you know too, is that the way you've been eating isn't working for you, and you need to change it! Specifically, you need to consume fewer calories than you have been. You also need to do a better job of timing your intake of those calories and making sure they are healthy ones. Fortunately, there are many diet options that can help you accomplish all of that.

What follows are a handful of diverse but proven dietary options you can choose from, based on your specific situation and individual preferences. I'm not a registered dietitian, but I don't have to be—hundreds of other people who *are* registered dietitians, medical doctors, or who hold PhDs have devised and/or scientifically tested some very good diets. What I'm doing here is giving you a synopsis of which ones merit further investigation on your part.

Your job is to read through my summaries of the different types of diets you might consider following and then pick one or a few to learn more about as you start to find your own ideal diet. I know, more work for you! Can't I just tell you which diet is the best one to follow? Okay, I will: the best diet for you is the one that gets you results *and that you will stick with for a lifetime*!

Of course, changing your way of eating is not going to be easy or quick. You'll need to put into practice every piece of information you learn by completing all of the exercises in this book in order to succeed. You'll stumble plenty of times and will need to backtrack and modify and forge a different course ahead. But even as you are struggling to find your ideal diet, you'll realize at points along the way just how far you've already come. "I can't believe I used to drink a six-pack of Coke every day!" you might say. Or, "Remember when all we ate for dinner were frozen entrées?" Or, "I haven't been to a fast-food restaurant in three months!" And those realizations will be monumental because they will represent significant, *permanent* behavior changes, which in turn will give you the confidence and motivation to continue making even more positive changes.

What follows is a short list of several different diets (by which I mean "ways of eating") that, if followed for the long term, will most certainly help you lose weight and keep it off. I'll tell you briefly what each plan entails, who it's intended for, its pros and cons, and I'll list at least one reference you can use to learn more about each one. Before I start, though, let me say that if you have been diagnosed with any chronic condition or precondition, if you are morbidly obese (your BMI is greater than 40), or if you have any food sensitivities or allergies, you MUST consult with a physician or registered dietitian before you implement any changes in your diet. Do not let this be a barrier to you! It is likely that your diet is the largest contributing factor to your current condition, so get the professional advice you need to start fixing yourself *right now*!

## DASH Eating Plan

The DASH (Dietary Approaches to Stop Hypertension) Eating Plan is recommended for people with high blood pressure (hypertension) or prehypertension. It has been shown to lower blood pressure and decrease the risk of heart disease in studies sponsored by the National Institutes of Health.[2] First and foremost, it is a low-salt (or, more accurately, low-sodium) plan, but it's also based on eating a diet rich in whole grains, fruits and vegetables, and low-fat or nonfat dairy. It is a high-fiber, low- to moderate-fat diet, rich in potassium, calcium, and magnesium. Learn more at http://www.nhlbi.nih.gov/health/health-topics/topics/dash/.

## American Diabetes Association Meal Plans

If you have been diagnosed with or are at risk for diabetes, you should definitely check out the ADA's meal plan website. It provides a lot of good information for just about any type of diet you want to follow. Some of the different meal plans covered include the plate method, carb counting, and using the glycemic index. The site also has extensive information on how to eat healthy if you want or need to follow a gluten-free or vegetarian diet. All of the different meal plans and methods discussed share the common goal of reducing risk of diabetes, and because BMI is highly correlated to risk for diabetes,[3] you can be sure that all of the dietary plans here are geared toward reaching and maintaining a healthy weight. Learn more at www.diabetes.org/food-and-fitness/.

## American Heart Association Dietary Guidelines

I am slightly less enamored with the American Heart Association's diet and lifestyle recommendations, primarily because they are pretty vague and don't lay out a specific list of foods with recommended number of servings. However, like the other dietary guideline sites, they do have some helpful online tools. If you go to the "Nutrition Center," you can find recipes, recommended cookbooks, a tool to help you make good choices when eating out, and another to help you plan meals and make a shopping list. If you've been diagnosed with heart disease or are at risk for developing it, this may be a good place for you to start. Find out more at www.heart.org (then click on "Getting Healthy" >"Nutrition Center").

## Whole-Food, Plant-Based Diet

On the face of it, this diet seems to be the most restrictive, as it is essentially a vegetarian or vegan diet that also limits *all* processed foods, including such favorites as flours and oils. In a way, though, that's also the beauty of it—as long as you load up on vegetables, fruits, legumes, and a few whole grains, nuts, and seeds, you can throw calorie counting out the window. The whole-food diet is inherently a low-calorie one because it eliminates such a large percentage of the high-calorie foods common in a Western diet (processed foods, high-fat animal-based foods, and foods with added sugars). Not only will you automatically reduce the "calories in" side of the equation, but research says this diet also boosts "calories out." One study found that thermogenesis, or the amount of calories needed to digest the food we eat, was nearly twice as high following a whole-foods meal than it was following one consisting of processed foods.[4] Proponents of this type of diet claim that absolutely no portion control or calorie counting is necessary. And that's the truth. If you faithfully stick to the list of "allowed" foods, you can pretty much eat all you want and you'll be likely to lose weight. The only potential trouble spots here are the whole grains and starches—the calories in those can add up quickly, but because you are limiting fat to a tiny amount and filling up on fruits and vegetables, grains and starches can be mixed into nearly every meal without thwarting your weight-loss efforts.

This diet is very high in fiber, vitamins, and minerals with the exception of vitamins D and B12, which you will need to supplement (many vegan foods are fortified with them, but you need to pay attention to daily intake levels). Researchers who have studied this diet have found it very effective not only for weight loss but for combating heart disease, high blood pressure, high cholesterol, and diabetes as well.[5] Somewhat surprisingly, they have also found that this diet is easier for participants to adopt and maintain than calorie-restricted diets.[6] While things like bread, pasta, boxed cereals, etc., are not part of the program, high-quality, whole-grain varieties of these premade foods are acceptable *occasionally*. Incidentally, a version of this diet was used by Dr. Ornish and colleagues in those groundbreaking epigenetic studies in 2008.

The biggest downside to this eating plan is that it requires you to do a lot of cooking, because packaged foods that meet these rigorous standards can be hard to find. Consumer demand for higher-quality convenience foods is on the rise, though, so there are more choices becoming available all the time. Just remember to ignore the marketing on the front of the package and scrutinize the nutrition label on the back to be sure you're getting a nutrient-dense meal and not a lot of empty calories.

Your best option, of course, is to cook your own food no matter which eating plan you choose. The quality of your meals and the amount of control you'll have over their nutritive value will more than make up for the time you spend in the kitchen. There are a number of very good resources to get you started online. Just type "whole foods plant based diet" into your favorite search engine.

## Mediterranen Diet

There are tons of websites, blogs, and books out there raving about the virtues of the Mediterranean (Med) Diet, but I like the way the Mayo Clinic outlines it on their website (see www.mayoclinic.com/health/mediterranean-diet/CL00011). At its heart, the Med Diet looks an awful lot like the Whole-Food, Plant-Based Diet, but it makes some allowances for non-plant-based foods and even recommends a little red wine! The key to this diet's success for weight loss lies in the *proportion* of the higher-fat and processed foods to the super-healthy whole grains, legumes, fruits, and vegetables. So don't think that because a little of something is included, a lot of it is acceptable!

If followed as intended, the Mediterranean Diet can not only help you lose weight, but it could also significantly reduce your risk of death due to heart disease and cancer.[7] Several studies have even shown a strong association between the Mediterranean Diet and a reduced risk of cognitive decline, including both Parkinson's and Alzheimer's diseases.[8]

The version of the Mediterranean Diet that produced these favorable research findings includes on average three or more servings per day of vegetables (excluding potatoes), two or more servings of fruit, one or more serving of whole grains and legumes, and around half a serving per day of fish and nuts or seeds. Red and/or processed meats should be limited to no more than four servings per week and mono- and polyunsaturated fats should be consumed in greater proportion than saturated fats. *Moderate* alcohol consumption of between 5 and 15 grams of alcohol by volume (that's only one cocktail, beer, or glass of wine) per day is also an optional part of the plan.[9]

## "Higher-Protein" Diet

Before you skip this section, thinking, "Been there, done that, hated it!" let me say that this is *not* a high-protein, low-carb diet. What I'm referring to with the "higher-protein" eating plan is a mountain of weight-loss research that has shown positive correlations between *moderately high* consumption of protein and weight loss. The studies found that protein consumption is linked to higher levels of satiety (you feel more full and satisfied) and thermogenesis (it takes more calories to process protein than fat or carbs), and it can help maintain muscle mass during weight loss and subsequent weight maintenance.[10]

But what constitutes "moderately high consumption," you ask? Well, it's somewhere around 30 percent of your total daily caloric intake. This should be your first clue that following the higher protein diet will require careful attention not only to calories consumed, but grams of protein, fat, and carbs as well. Simply trying to "get more protein" into your diet can easily backfire, causing you to consume more total calories if you don't adjust the amount of fat and carbohydrates downward. Also, be very aware that many foods considered to be "high protein" are actually "high fat." Many meats, dairy products, eggs, and nuts can have as many or more of their calories derived from fat than from protein.

Notably, the successful weight-management trials involving higher protein consumption kept fat intake at or below 20 percent of calories. This leaves you able to consume around 50 percent of your calories from carbohydrates, which is a far cry from the brand-name, low-carb fad diets on the market.

If you're interested in seeing whether more protein can make a difference for you, I recommend you have a registered dietitian make a personalized plan for you. If you'd rather go it alone, you can start by choosing one of the other eating plans discussed above as a general guide, and then add in more of your favorite lean protein sources to get you to the target percentage. Just be sure you are cutting the same number of calories from the fat and/or carbohydrate categories so that you don't exceed your daily calorie goal. (If you're going the higher-protein, plant-based route, then you won't need to count calories once you've completed the remaining food log exercises in the chapters ahead.)

## Hey, I Think I See a Trend Here!

Not surprisingly, there are some things that all of these diets have in common. They all limit saturated fats. They emphasize fruits, vegetables, legumes, and whole grains. They limit consumption of processed or highly refined foods and ingredients (white bread, white pasta, table sugar, corn syrup, etc.), and recommend limiting sodium. So in general, a healthy diet that will result in weight loss does *not* include fast food, fried foods, baked goods or other sugary desserts, fatty red or processed meats, high-fat cheese (and especially not "processed cheese food"), ice cream, whole milk, cream, butter, margarine, or more than two daily servings of any oil.

## 5 Simple Rules

Finding the right eating plan for *you* will be essential to the success of your weight-loss effort. While dieting can seem overwhelming with so many choices and so much misleading marketing, there are actually a few simple guidelines that will put you on the right path and help you make better dietary choices, regardless of which eating plan you choose to follow. I will give you many useful tips and tricks for healthy eating later, in chapter 11, but to get you started, here are my five simple rules for healthy eating:

1. Choose Whole Foods.
2. Eat More Plants.
3. Make *All* of Your Snacks Healthy Ones.
4. Don't Drink Your Calories.
5. Choose Protein Sources with Two Legs or Fewer.

First, always opt for whole foods over processed ones. If a food still looks like it did when it was growing, you'll be getting the maximum nutrients and fiber from it and a limited amount of added sugar, fat, and preservatives. Whole foods are generally lower in calories and are always of higher nutritive quality than their packaged and processed counterparts. Eating whole foods doesn't have to mean eating them raw, but choose the healthiest method of preparation that makes them palatable to you. For vegetables, this means steaming, baking, boiling, or lightly sautéing in a nonstick pan lined with a bit of water, broth, or a tiny amount of oil. For fish, poultry, and meats, grilling is your best option, but roasting and stewing are good options too. If you have to add sugar, butter, salt, sauces, or loads of dressing to a food to make it taste good, then you should leave it out of your diet and opt for other foods instead.

Second, the more plant based your diet is, the better. Not only are plant-based foods nearly always lower in calories and fat than their animal-based counterparts, but plants contain loads of vitamins, minerals, antioxidants, and fiber, so they are super healthy too. Of course, there is plenty of plant-based junk food out there, so be sure that you apply Rule #1 before you apply Rule #2! Put simply, you should aim for four to five servings of raw or healthfully prepared vegetables and two or three servings of fruit every day.

Rule #3 can be tough to stick to, and you probably won't all the time, but if you remember the rule and apply it as often as possible, you'll end up cutting out a lot of empty calories throughout the day. Rather than having a cookie or a sweet roll or half a bag of chips when you're feeling snacky, if you opt instead for an apple, some fresh pineapple, or an ounce of lightly salted nuts you'll be helping yourself out in two ways. First, you'll be replacing an unhealthy, empty-calorie snack with a healthier one that is also probably lower in calories. Second, you'll be breaking the emotional "food as reward" system you had in place before. By eating junk food whenever you're bored, tired, stressed, depressed, or in association with certain activities, you've built up strong pathways making these choices almost automatic. Train yourself to select from among healthy options instead, and suddenly you've made eating a snack more about fueling your body and less about satisfying some emotional want.

Rule #4: I'll harp on this again in chapter 11, but it bears mentioning now because so many people consume so many of their calories from beverages. On the face of it, this should be an easy way to shed anywhere from 50 to 500 calories from your diet every day, but beverages are tricky characters in many of our lives. Whether it's the regular mid-morning coffee drink with whipped cream and chocolate sauce, a favorite soda, beer, wine, or cocktails, many people have a preferred high-calorie beverage that they drink ritually for emotional or social reasons. Another problem is that beverages are heavily marketed to us, making it more difficult to resist their tempting lure. You should have learned from your initial week of food logging whether beverages constitute a calorie concern for you. If they do, be mindful of this and look for ways to wean yourself away from them.

Rule #5 can be a controversial one. There is much heated debate among various dietary camps over the topic of protein and its best sources. While vegans rail against protein from *any* animal source, paleo-enthusiasts argue just the opposite—that man has evolved to favor animal flesh as the most viable form of protein. Ethical considerations and personal preferences aside, there are a few indisputable facts that have led me to the creation of Rule #5.

First, there are only two commonly eaten plant sources that qualify as "complete" proteins, providing the proper proportions of all the essential amino acids the human body needs. These are soy and quinoa. (It should be noted, however, that one of the amino acids in quinoa is present at a level lower than is required by humans, so often soy is the only plant given this distinction.) It's easy to get all of the essential amino acids when eating a variety of plant sources, but generally speaking, plants contain lower levels of protein than animal sources do.

On the flip side, animal sources of protein often come with a lot of unwanted baggage. Higher fat (and especially saturated fat) content is one, and dietary cholesterol is another. Not only that, but some farm animals are given hormones to speed their growth, and many are administered antibiotics to help them survive the less-than-optimal conditions on large farms. A label on your meat stating that no hormones were used is pretty trustworthy, but there is wide variation and little oversight when it comes to antibiotics.

So, in order to arrive at a healthy, higher-protein, lower-fat diet, I've found that a pretty easy rule of thumb is to count the number of legs on your source of protein. It's hard to do better than fish for a source of lean protein *as long as your fish came from a decent place.* Opt for wild-caught rather than farmed fish, and try to stick with those caught in the United States or Canada. Chicken, turkey, or other poultry are pretty good protein options too, with white meat having lower levels of saturated fat and cholesterol. An occasional lean cut of beef, lamb, or pork is fine, but it's very easy for calories from fat to skyrocket when four-legged animals are on your table. Even "90% lean" ground beef has around one-third more fat and nearly twice as much saturated fat as ground turkey.

In terms of plants, legumes (especially lentils) are protein powerhouses, and very high in fiber too. Pairing beans with a whole grain (like brown rice or quinoa) will supply all of the essential amino acids and very little fat with zero cholesterol. Eggs and low-fat or fat-free dairy are pretty good choices too. Just mind the cholesterol in the eggs and maybe toss out the yolks if it's a concern for you. Also, watch for added sugars in low-fat and fat-free dairy products, especially yogurt and flavored milks.

Remember, too, that the way your protein source is prepared can turn something reasonably healthy into a fat and calorie disaster. Avoid breaded and fried meats or those served with rich sauces or added fat from pan drippings. Finally, avoid cured and processed meats (bacon, sausage, and hot dogs) like the plague! They are ultra high in fat, cholesterol, and calories, and most contain nitrates (which have been linked to certain forms of cancer) and off-the-charts levels of sodium.

## Put Together Your Own Best Diet

Regardless of which eating plan you choose, it's important to acknowledge now that this effort is going to require you to make changes to the way you eat. Depending on your current eating habits, you might need to make quite a few changes that are pretty large in scope. While no food has to be totally off-limits forever, if you are to be successful, you'll need to limit your servings of those high-calorie, low-nutrient foods to one or two per *week*, and I'm sorry to say that's a combined total—not one or two servings of each!

You might be wondering what's left that you *can* eat on a regular basis. Well, everything else, of course! There are plenty of good food choices remaining, and there are tens of thousands of resources in print and online to help you build an arsenal of health-boosting, fat-shedding recipes. There is just one catch, one potentially big obstacle you're going to have to overcome: What if you don't really like any of that healthy stuff? The bad news is, to lose weight and keep it off, you have to eat the healthy stuff. The good news is, we are *all* physiologically capable of changing our tastes—but more on that later. For now, you have some work to do.

## ⊘ Exercise 13: Pick a Diet, Any Diet!

Now it's time to roll up your sleeves and get down to business. After reading the information above, you might already be certain which eating plan you'd like to follow, or you might have several that you need to learn more about before making your decision.

If you're telling yourself, "I'm just going to eat healthier. I'll cut out X, Y, and Z and that should do the trick," then you could be setting yourself up for failure. It is true that the worse your eating habits are now, the more successful this strategy could be. If you routinely eat pizza, burgers, or fried foods and drink a lot of high-caloric beverages, it is actually possible to have great early success just by cutting out these "worst offenders." But know that any success you enjoy will be short-lived if that's all you do. Eventually you will need to truly change your eating habits. So for this exercise I'm asking you to put in the effort to select the healthy eating plan you'd like to try following. At this point, you don't even have to make any radical changes if you're not ready. Just explore your options, do the research, and commit to a plan that you're willing to call "My Eating Plan." Outline, in great detail, what that plan looks like. Get specific about the types of food you'll try to eat more of, the types you'll try to eat less of, and what you're going to try cutting out entirely.

I urge you not to be overly restrictive with your initial diet plan. If you choose a diet that has you eating only foods that you hate, you won't stick with it. It's okay to choose a plan that's a compromise between what you consider ideal for weight loss and what you consider easy to follow. After you've come up with your diet, we'll focus on implementing a few healthy changes in Exercise 14, but for now, this is a planning exercise only.

## Character Example

After reading over the list of diets, Ellen has a couple in mind that she wants to explore further. She checks out a number of websites with information about the Mediterranean diet and browses the American Diabetes Association's website. She also goes to the local bookstore and leafs through about twenty different cookbooks that seem to fall under the "healthy" category. She writes the following in her notebook:

*Exercise 13: My Diet*

*After doing a lot of research, I've chosen the Mediterranean diet as the model for how I want to eat. I thought about the whole-foods, plant-based diet, but I think I would miss chicken and fish too much. I did buy a vegetarian cookbook that had a lot of great-looking recipes, though. Here's how I will define my diet:*

*General Description: This diet is primarily plant-based, with a moderate amount of lean animal protein like fish, poultry, low-fat dairy, and eggs. Saturated fat is very limited, and healthy fats from plant sources are emphasized, though in small quantities.*

*Foods I Will Eat More Of:*
- *Vegetables—try to get in a big variety, especially leafy greens*
- *Legumes*
- *Fish*
- *Fruits*
- *Nuts and seeds (1 serving daily)*
- *Lean poultry (less frequently)*
- *Whole grains*
- *Healthy oils (no more than 2 tablespoons daily)*

*Foods I Will Eat Less Of:*
- *Processed carbohydrates (bread, pasta, white rice)*
- *Sugar—all forms!*
- *Red meat*

*Foods I Will Cut Out Entirely:*
- *Processed meats*
- *Fried foods*

## Putting Your Dietary Plan into Practice

Now that you've chosen your dietary guidelines and laid out the ground rules for yourself, you'll need to set up a framework for measuring how well you follow your plan. I hate to say it, but here comes the food log again.

In the following exercise, you will identify which eating behaviors you want to change first. It is imperative, however, that at this point you *don't set a goal of limiting your calories to a specific number.* I know I've been harping on the importance of calories, and now I'm telling you to forget about that for a while. The trouble is, if you focus on the numbers right now, you're likely to sabotage yourself. Because you haven't learned your new healthy eating behaviors yet, you'll likely fall into the "diet" trap again if you simply try to downsize your current diet to fit a lower-calorie target.

## A Calorie Is a Calorie, or Not

Over and over again I've seen clients fall into the pit of calorie counting. They log their food and exercise, tracking their calories in and out, and despite my constant warnings and protestations, they become fixated on the numbers and try to "game" the system. And the scale does not budge for them. "How can this be?!" they ask, thinking that if they can somehow make their net calories at the end of every day fall around 500 to the negative, they will "automatically" lose a pound per week.

In theory, this should happen. But only if the theory is backed up by flawless calorie tracking, and only if the calories they're consuming don't negatively affect their metabolism. These people have forgotten about (or choose to ignore) all of the built-in inaccuracies with calorie tracking, and they're not listening when I tell them that a calorie is not always a calorie and they need to focus on quality as well as quantity. These clients are the Savers—they skimp on nutrients and "save calories" throughout the day so they can splurge later, "spending" those calories on alcoholic beverages, big dinners, or fattening desserts. They feel tired and sluggish throughout the day due to a lack of quality fuel coming in, and they sabotage their body's chance for a good night's sleep by giving it too much to digest when it should be resting and rejuvenating. Their workouts suffer, they are irritable, and when the scale doesn't reflect what they were hoping to see, they grow frustrated and give up altogether.

Consider this: It takes about twice as many calories for the body to digest and process a gram of protein as it does to process a gram of carbohydrate, and between *six and ten times as much as* a gram of fat.[11] Also fiber, being largely indigestible, uses up half of the calories it possesses.[12] Add to this the fact that a gram of fat contains more than twice as many calories as a gram of protein, and you can see how quickly the numbers can stack against you. This is why some people can seemingly eat all the time while others are "starving" themselves, yet the healthy eaters lose weight more quickly because their *net* calorie total is lower. So two people eating a diet of the same *number* of calories, but calories of different *types*, can experience very different outcomes in terms of how those calories are processed by the body. "Empty-calorie" diets high in fat and sugar disrupt the metabolism and lead to weight gain.[13]

Imagine Person A, who eats a nutrient-dense, high-fiber, higher-protein diet loaded with fruits, vegetables, and whole grains, and who limits saturated fat and added sugars. She is giving her body a constant supply of high-quality energy, and she feels fuller throughout the day even though she may be eating fewer calories than she used to. In contrast, Person B skips breakfast so she can have a high-fat, sugary coffee drink mid-morning, then has a tiny frozen diet entrée for lunch and a big dinner high in fat and refined carbohydrates (e.g., pasta Alfredo, bread, and wine). At the end of the day, she's happy to see that she has a few hundred calories "to spare" (which is probably a farce due to inaccurate food logging), so she eats half a chocolate bar or has another glass of wine before bedtime. All throughout the day, Person B feels hungry and her energy peaks and plummets. At the end of the day she feels that she really deserves her "treat" because she has "followed her diet" so well when, in fact, she is sabotaging her metabolism and compromising all of her body's systems. It's only a matter of time before she falls ill or begins to experience negative gastric or other consequences from this way of eating. She is suffering need- lessly, all for a few minutes of gratification at the end of a very long day. This is why, at this point, you must focus on behaviors and types of food only, and not on calories.

##  Exercise 14: Start to Change the Way You Eat.

It's time to put your new dietary plan into action. For this exercise, look at the prelimi- nary one-week food log you kept in Exercise 6 and see how your current diet differs most from your chosen new diet. Write down the two or three most obvious things you'd like to change about your old ways of eating. Next, specifically say *how* you will transform those two or three old, negative habits into two or three positive habits that are in line with your new way of eating. These should be specific dietary behaviors—actionable steps that you can take every day—that will become healthy eating habits when maintained over time. It's fine (desirable, even) to observe the effect that changing these behaviors has on your daily calorie totals, but the overall goal right now should not be calculated calorie restriction.

## Character Example

Cindy reviews her original seven-day food log, including the notes she wrote each day and the summary notes from the end of her first week of logging. Right away she can see two big changes she could make that would pay big dividends. Cindy has decided to try out the whole-foods, plant-based eating plan. She gets out her notebook and writes:

*Exercise 14: Start to Change the Way I Eat.*

*After reading about the way I should be eating and looking further into the whole-foods, plant-based way of eating, I know I have a lot of changes to make. To get started, though, I'm going to focus on just the two things that I think are hurting me the most:*

1. *I get too many calories from beverages. If I did nothing but cut out those creamy, sweetened coffee drinks, the juice that I thought was healthy, and happy-hour drinks, I could lose a pound a week! I don't think I can be that drastic, though, so here's what I'll do: I will stop getting those high-calorie coffee drinks and have regular coffee with 1 tablespoon of cream and 1 sugar instead. I'll quit drinking the juice and have a piece of fruit or some raw veggies instead and will drink water with my lunch. I'll limit myself to four alcoholic drinks per week.*

2. *I never eat breakfast at home, but I'm always hungry in the morning. This means I either hit the drive-through on the way into work or get a pastry from the coffee shop around the corner. These are poor food choices resulting in tons of empty calories, and they don't even make me feel that full, so I often eat again mid-morning (usually another sugary, fat-filled snack). I will commit to eating a decent breakfast at home every morning.*

Once you've decided which eating behaviors to modify, you'll need to set up a way to measure your progress. Resume logging your food in order to do this. It's also time to take your food log a step further and select the other parameters you want to measure, such as percent of calories from fat, grams of sugars, etc. In this exercise you will use your food log not only to track what you eat but also as a tool to help shape your behaviors. It will help tremendously if you start preplanning your meals and snacks with your first dietary behavior changes in mind.

At this point, if you must, you can plug in the number of pounds per week you want to lose. I recommend that you enter no more than one-half pound per week, *and I stress again the importance of not focusing primarily on calories!* I promise we'll get to that part when the time is right, but for now you should be using your food log to monitor how successfully you implement your first few behavior changes.

## ✐ Exercise 15: Measure Your Progress.

I recommend that at this point you decide which dietary nutrients you want to track and keep track of those in your food log. Most programs will automatically calculate grams of protein, fat, and carbohydrates for you, and many will give you a chart or report of what percentage of your daily calories come from each of those, but you'll often have the option to choose one or two other nutrients to track. Pick those things you are most concerned with. If you eat a lot of sugar, then track grams of sugar. If you have high blood pressure, you may want to keep track of sodium. If you're at risk for heart disease, then you'll want to limit saturated fat, so keep tabs on that. Of course, if you're using pen and paper or some other nonautomated method, then you can track whatever you want; you'll just have to spend a little more time tabulating everything yourself.

## Character Example

We'll look in on Cindy again, because you're familiar with her original seven-day food log and she's just told us which behaviors she wants to change.

*Exercise 15: Measure Your Progress.*

*This week I'm going to eat a healthy breakfast at home every day and drastically reduce my calories from beverages. Since I'm trying out the whole-foods, plant-based diet, I'm a little worried about getting enough protein, so I definitely want to track that. I also want to be sure I'm getting a lot less sugar and saturated fat than before because I know that's where most of my empty calories are coming from.*

Cindy enters the following parameters into her food log program. She is only using this food log to track diet, not exercise, so she has told the program not to count exercise by entering zeros into those fields. I recommend that you do the same (more about why in the next chapter). Note also that she has still told the program she is only trying to maintain weight. She does this so that she's not tempted to be overly concerned with cutting calories.

| Personal Information | | | |
|---|---|---|---|
| Current Weight: | 192 lbs. | | |
| Goal Weight: | 150 lbs. | | |
| Height: | 5 ft. | 8 in. | |
| Gender: | male | X female | |
| Date of Birth: | September | 1 | 1985 |
| Normal Daily Activity Level | | | |
| X Sedentary | Spend most of the day sitting (e.g. bank teller, desk job) | | |
| Somewhat Active | Spend a good part of the day on your feet (e.g. teacher, salesman) | | |
| Active | Spend a good part of the day doing some physical activity (e.g. waitress, mailman) | | |
| Very Active | Spend most of the day doing heavy physical activity (e.g. bike messenger, carpenter) | | |
| Exercise | | | |
| Weekly Goal | 0 workouts/week | 0 minutes/workout | |
| Preferred Tracking | X Calories | Kilojoules | |
| Goal | | | |
| What is your goal? | Maintain my current weight | | |
| Nutrients Tracked | | | |
| X | Calories (required) | | |
| X | Carbohydrates | | |
| X | Fat | | |
| X | Protein | | |
| X | Sugar | | |
| X | Saturated Fat | | |

Cindy spends the next week carefully tracking everything she eats and drinks. She's not changing her whole diet right away; she's just working on breakfast and beverages. Because she's chosen the whole-foods, plant-based diet, she plans and shops for breakfast items that fall within those guidelines. She starts ordering her coffee with nondairy creamer, but she doesn't worry much at all about the other snacks and meals of the day. When she's presented with options that easily fall into her new eating plan, she chooses them, but her main focus for this week is changing those first two dietary behaviors. Here's what a sample day from her food log looks like:

| Breakfast | Quantity | Calories | Carbs | Fat | Protein | Sugar | Sat Fat |
|---|---|---|---|---|---|---|---|
| Organic Old-fashioned Oats | ½ cup | 150 | 27 | 3 | 5 | 0 | 1 |
| Banana | 1 small, 101g | 90 | 23 | 0 | 1 | 12 | 0 |
| Almond Milk | 1 cup | 30 | 4 | 1 | 1 | 4 | 0 |
| Coffee, brewed from grounds | 2 cups | 5 | 0 | 0 | 1 | 0 | 0 |
| Sugar, natural cane turbinado | 1 tsp | 15 | 4 | 0 | 0 | 4 | 0 |
| Creamer, nondairy | 1 tsp | 10 | 2 | 0 | 0 | 0 | 0 |
| Walnuts, chopped | 10g | 65 | 0 | 6 | 2 | 0 | 0 |
| | Totals | 365 | 60 | 10 | 10 | 20 | 1 |
| Lunch | Quantity | Calories | Carbs | Fat | Protein | Sugar | Sat Fat |
| Veggie Sub (Alto) | 6 inch | 400 | 71 | 9 | 9 | 5 | 5 |
| Carbonated Water (Streamz) | 12 oz. | 0 | 0 | 0 | 0 | 0 | 0 |
| Potato Chips (Chloe's) | 1 oz. | 150 | 15 | 10 | 2 | 1 | 3 |
| | Totals | 550 | 86 | 19 | 11 | 6 | 8 |
| Dinner | Quantity | Calories | Carbs | Fat | Protein | Sugar | Sat Fat |
| Burrito, bean and cheese | 1 burrito | 378 | 55 | 12 | 15 | 0 | 7 |
| Guacamole, mild | 2 tbsp | 29 | 4 | 1 | 0 | 0 | 0 |
| Beer, lager | 12 oz. | 145 | 0 | 0 | 0 | 0 | 0 |
| Rice, white medium-grained | 1 cup | 242 | 53 | 0 | 4 | 0 | 0 |
| Chocolate Cake (Coco's) | 1/3 slice | 219 | 24 | 13 | 3 | 14 | 8 |
| | Totals | 1,013 | 136 | 26 | 22 | 14 | 15 |
| Snacks | Quantity | Calories | Carbs | Fat | Protein | Sugar | Sat Fat |
| Pineapple, raw fresh | 1 cup, 165 g | 82 | 22 | 0 | 1 | 16 | 0 |
| Chocolate Chip Cookies | 1 oz. | 130 | 17 | 7 | 1 | 0 | 2 |
| Creamer, nondairy | 1 tsp | 10 | 2 | 0 | 0 | 0 | 0 |
| Sugar, natural cane turbinado | 1 tsp | 15 | 4 | 0 | 0 | 4 | 0 |
| Coffee, brewed from grounds | 2 cups | 5 | 0 | 0 | 1 | 0 | 0 |
| | Totals | 242 | 45 | 7 | 3 | 20 | 2 |
| | | Calories | Carbs | Fat | Protein | Sugar | Sat Fat |
| | Daily | 2,170 | 327 | 62 | 46 | 60 | 26 |
| | Daily Goal | 2,060 | 258 | 69 | 103 | 77 | 23 |

*I went out with the girls tonight—big dinner! It was hard to limit myself to one beer, but I did it! I really wanted a glass of wine with dessert. I like the oatmeal with banana and walnuts for breakfast, and I'm getting used to the almond milk. I'm still not a big fan of the nondairy creamer. Maybe I'll try the almond milk in my coffee tomorrow. Cutting out the juice has been easy. I do miss my fancy coffee drink mid-morning, but I'm okay with getting a regular coffee. I still had a cookie with it today, though. That might be the next thing I try to work on. I'd also like to try to get a little more protein. So far, though, I'm doing really well with my first two behaviors. I missed breakfast at home one morning, but they actually serve a hot whole-grain cereal at the coffee shop—who knew?! The oatmeal I make at home is way better, though (and doesn't cost $5), so that's only a backup. My average daily calories for this week were so much lower than for the week before—I feel like this weight-loss thing might actually be possible!*

It's important to notice a few things from Cindy's example. First, her behavior-change goals were very realistic. They were things that had the potential to make a big impact, but she was careful not to make them radically restrictive. She didn't dictate exactly what she would eat every morning, for example, only that it would be "healthier" and that it would follow her whole-foods, plant-based diet. She also didn't say that she would stop drinking coffee or alcohol altogether, and she offered herself an alternative to the juice (whole fruit or veggies).

The second thing to notice is that Cindy wasn't perfect, but she was flexible. When she missed breakfast at home, she didn't allow herself to get a donut or muffin, but instead, she chose a very close substitute for her at-home breakfast.

Most importantly, Cindy isn't getting bogged down in the numbers at this point. She's making some observations about them, but for this whole week, she has focused on her two key behaviors.

## A Little Help

Behavior change is difficult, even if you're only changing a couple of relatively small things at a time. Here's a little insight that might make the process a bit easier for you.

It's all well and good to know which diet you want to follow and which bad habits you want to change first, but how do you go about successfully implementing those changes without falling into old diet traps? For each person there's a slightly different process or formula, and the approach you take to finding yours depends primarily on your personality type.

Some people just want to be told what to do. If Cindy were that type of person, she might have planned out exactly what she was going to eat for breakfast every day and stuck to that schedule as though it were law. She also might have decided that it would be easier to forbid drinking alcohol completely than to allow herself a few drinks over the course of a week. Most of us are not that way—we rail against the idea of all-or-nothing restriction and would rebel against ourselves if we made such stringent rules. But it's important to know which type of person you are, because the *way* you set your goals can be as important as what those goals entail.

If you don't care to follow a regimented plan, then use your food log to make gradual changes daily. Each night review your log and assess how the day went. Look for positives and areas for improvement, and commit to doing a little better the next day. This is a learning process, not a trial by fire. Be firm with yourself, but also be a bit forgiving and, above all, be flexible. If you can't make a perfect choice, make the next best choice. Consistent and gradual improvement is what you're after.

*This is how behavior change works—incrementally,*
*with small successes building upon small successes,*
*until their sum becomes hugely effective.*

Remember also that at every stage of this process, *your attitude and your intentions will define your level of success.* If you approach your dietary behavior changes with the same negative attitude you've had in the past, you will have exactly the same results as before. If, however, you approach these changes with a new excitement and clearly stated intentions, then you can expect to radically change the way you interact with food. The key is to remain laser focused on only those behaviors you are working on at the current stage and to keep your motivation high across all stages.

Okay, it's time to move on from diet to exercise. We'll get into greater detail about setting your daily calorie target a bit later, but for now, keep working on your first few dietary behaviors until they become second nature.

## Chapter Five

# EXERCISE: MOVE OR DIE

In the press, diet nearly always gets top billing when it comes to weight loss, while exercise is often downplayed, disregarded, or sometimes even spurned. It makes some sense, considering that many solid studies have shown that exercise *alone* does not lead to significant weight loss. But the main reason for this is pretty straightforward: while exercise is a great way to create a calorie deficit, running low on calories causes you to be hungry, which causes you to eat more. Interestingly, though, research has shown that exercise itself does not increase appetite, but in many cases suppresses it.[1] It is the ongoing calorie deficit that increases hunger and leads to compensatory eating. This deficit could just as easily be created by calorie restriction alone, but the reason why exercise alone performs worse against diet alone in weight loss is largely psychological in nature:[2] if you're relying on exercise alone and ignoring the dietary component, when you feel hungry you'll eat more. You may do this without even realizing it, or you might tell yourself that you "deserve" a bigger meal, an unplanned snack, or a high-calorie treat because you worked so hard in the gym. Unfortunately, this erases your calorie deficit, and the scale doesn't budge. Put simply, if you aren't paying attention to both parts of the calories in–calories out formula, then all your time spent exercising might amount to wasted effort. The good news is that a large body of scientific evidence says that *adding* exercise to a sound dietary strategy is by far the most effective way to lose weight.[3]

Perhaps the most exciting and compelling case for exercise comes from a 2013 epigenetic study published in the online journal *PLOS Genetics*. In it, researchers found that a six-month exercise program favorably altered the genetic expression of fat cells in thirty-nine genes thought to be associated with obesity and type 2 diabetes.[4] Here is concrete proof that lifestyle intervention does change the body at the cellular level!

Still, many people choose to skip the exercise component, opting instead to lose their weight through diet alone. Some of them do lose a significant amount of weight, but few of them will keep the weight off. While exercise plays a small but significant role in the weight-loss process, studies have found it to be all but essential for keeping the weight off once it's been lost.[5] Not only that, but exercise also has a profoundly positive effect on body composition (the ratio of fat mass to lean muscle mass), irrespective of weight loss.[6]

Nobody wants to hear about tiny amounts of weight loss or positive changes in body composition without weight loss, but think about this: What if you had been maintaining your weight over the past one, five, or twenty years by building a little muscle and losing a little fat instead of the other way around? You probably wouldn't be reading this book, I'm guessing.

So exercise *is* important to the weight-loss process in terms of the calorie equation, but it also provides many other benefits that can accelerate your weight loss. Exercise improves mood, boosts energy, helps you sleep better, lowers blood sugar and cholesterol levels, improves range of motion and joint fluidity, combats hypertension and atherosclerosis, and improves balance, agility, and coordination.[7]

The human body was designed to move. That's why we are upright, bi-pedal animals. Our bodies were not designed to sit at a desk all day or (worse) to slouch half propped up in bed or on a couch for hours every evening. The fact that people habitually do these things now is the obvious reason why many are overweight. We experience fatigue and pain, irritability and depression, stiffness of our joints, and a softness of our musculature. And exercise is the only remedy for these things. Why, then, are you not eagerly jumping out of your chair to do it right now?

Step Eight:

# START MOVING EVERY DAY

## Overcoming Inertia

"A body at rest tends to stay at rest . . ." I'm certain that Sir Isaac Newton wasn't referring to human bodies when he wrote his First Law of Motion, but it is applicable today, isn't it? We humans are creatures of habit and comfort, and we find it generally cozy and easy to sit around doing nothing. But having made the case for exercise above, let's spend some time looking at how you can overcome your own inertia.

If you don't currently exercise at all, then you're in luck, for you will have the biggest potential gains to realize from beginning an exercise regimen. Of course, getting to the point where you're doing it regularly for the rest of your life is another matter.

If you currently exercise every once in a while, then that's a good place to start, and we can work on creating a routine. If you already exercise regularly, then good for you—completing the next exercise will be a breeze! In any case, before we get to the next exercise, let me help you get some potential excuses out of the way.

## Common Excuses for Not Exercising

*I'm embarrassed.*

If you are currently sedentary (perhaps you've *never* exercised, or at least not since you were forced to do it in gym class), then you might have some strong emotional issues regarding your dislike of physical activity. Many people have felt awkward and/or were made fun of by others in school because they were "not athletic." (Let me take this opportunity to suggest to those of you who have school-aged children of your own to intervene now, while you can, so that they neither suffer the same fate as you, nor subject others to similar poor treatment.)

I understand the powerful impact that these experiences can have on a person, even decades later. But what you must come to understand (and quickly) is that you are no longer a child in school, and adults are generally a lot nicer to one another than children are. Also, performance is no longer an issue for you. No one is picking you for a team, no one is competing against you at exercise, and probably they aren't even comparing themselves to you. So if you feel awkward donning your exercise clothes and going out into the world, there are two things you should know: (1) it's normal for you to feel that way; and (2) no one is really looking at you, so get over it.

You may weigh 400 or 500 pounds. People may stare at you when you walk down the sidewalk. You probably imagine all sorts of horrible things they're thinking or whispering about you. But probably they're just worried about getting to where they need to be on time. Sure, there are some people who judge others, and a few of them may be cruel, but they're not likely to be members of the same gym as you. I myself can be a bit judgmental (but mostly sad) when I see a very overweight person participating in behaviors that are contributing to their unhealthy condition; however, I have nothing but admiration for a very overweight person who is out there on a walking path, a treadmill, or circuit-training machines.

If you simply can't overcome your fear of judgment by others, then you'll have to spend a little money to outfit your home with some basic exercise equipment and do your workouts there, in an environment you consider safe. But I urge you to at least consider this a temporary measure. Once you've lost a bit of weight and feel more comfortable with exercise, consider joining a gym or an activity group. There are a few reasons why this is important. First, it's a bigger commitment on your part, so it adds another layer of accountability. If you're a regular at your gym or in a walking group and you miss a few days, people might ask where you've been. This will encourage you not to miss as many days. Second, exercise should be as fun and as social as you can make it. For all but the most die-hard loners, doing an activity with a group is much more rewarding than doing the same activity alone. Even just lifting weights in a gym among a few other people you don't know can give you a social experience and a sense of camaraderie—you are in a place doing an activity with like-minded individuals, no matter how different your fitness and ability levels may be. Finally, you'll have access to many different types of (and likely much higher-quality) equipment at a gym than you can afford or fit into your home. You will understand the benefit of access to more equipment when I discuss how it's important to change up your workout routine every couple of months later in chapter 10.

### I don't have time.

Here's a common one: "I'm so busy, I don't have any time to exercise." Everyone says it and everyone is on Facebook or watching the latest HBO series or carting their kids off to twelve different after-school activities every day. My point is that certain discretionary activities could be replaced with exercise. What you need to do is ask yourself which of those activities are more important than your health.

I don't know about you, but I don't think I've ever "found" a chunk of time lying around in the middle of my day, available for me to do whatever I want with it since, oh, sixth grade. Our days are full of activity *because we design them to be.* We fill our days with things that fall into three categories: things we have to do, should do, and want to do. For those who lead happy, balanced lives, there's a good mix of all three woven into each day.

For each of us, exercise falls into one of those three categories, depending on our own personal attitude toward it. I would argue that if you can successfully place it into the "have to" category, then you're more likely to get your workouts in nearly every day. By giving exercise the priority it deserves and moving it out of the discretionary pile, you'll be much less likely to let it slip off your daily schedule when things get hectic.

If you can start viewing your workouts as protected time that's just for you—time that you know makes you better in every way—and if you can find a few activities that really make you enjoy that time, then you can place your workouts in the "want to" category, and the chances of exercise becoming a daily habit are quite high. This is where finding an activity you love, or incorporating a social aspect into your workouts, can pay big dividends.

If you view exercise as something you "should" do, then you have an uphill battle on your hands. I can't count the number of things I should do every day but don't. I should floss twice a day, I should dust the bookshelves, I should eat broccoli, and I should take a continuing education course. But I ignore most of these things until they become "have to's." The "should do's" will likely end up eliminated first when something unexpected comes up in your day, and something unexpected always comes up. Exercise cannot be one of those things—it's too important for that!

I'll tell you why you should view exercise as something you have to do every day: it's your duty. Exercise improves mood, cardiovascular and muscular function, immune system function, energy levels, and mental acuity, and you owe it to everyone around you to keep all those things running smoothly. You know that all-important job you devote so much of your time to? Even if there is not the slightest trace of a physical aspect to it, you could be doing it much better if you were alert, in a good mood, and full of energy.

Think about how much more you could offer your family if you were healthier. What kind of a spouse/partner/parent/son/daughter are you right now? What kind of contributions do you make to the family unit? Do you bring a sense of vibrancy home each evening, or do you struggle just to deal with everything that's going on? Are you a drain on other family members because you're often sick, tired, crabby, or stressed? Wouldn't you rather be a healthy, energetic, and positive role model for those around you?

So, basically, if you have *anyone* else at all in your life who depends on you, even a little—if you are a teacher, manager, peer-to-peer trainer, mentor, or team member; if you are a parent, grandparent, son or daughter, sibling, spouse or partner; if you are a volunteer, friend, or neighbor—then you owe it to everyone to become a more positive, healthy individual and start contributing at a higher level. And that is why you *have to* exercise!

So stop trying to "find" time to exercise. There isn't any time to find. You need to *make* the time, every day. It needs to be a non-optional, automatic activity that's simply part of your day. It needs to stop being the first "negotiable" thing that's eliminated when your schedule runs tight. It needs to be like brushing your teeth or taking a shower or paying the electric bill on time. In a real emergency, you can skip these things once in a great while, but start skipping them on a regular basis, and the negative impacts can be clearly seen and felt. It's just like that with exercise—if you let it go for far too long, you're forced to deal with the negative consequences.

### But I hate it!

Finally, there will be many of you out there who just plain hate to exercise, and that's your reason for not doing it. All I can say is, I'm right there with you. For me, exercise falls somewhere on the enjoyability scale between brushing my teeth and scooping the cat litter. These are not things one does for fun, but rather because not doing them over time results in negative consequences. I will admit that there are some forms of exercise I truly enjoy—a bike ride on a beautiful summer day, an easy jog down along the river or through a beautiful park, a relaxing yoga session—but for the most part, my aim is to do it and get it done so I can get on with the more pleasant aspects of my day. Really, that's about the best most of us can expect. But there are a couple of things you can try that will make exercise as enjoyable as possible, even if you never learn to truly love it.

The most important thing you can do is avoid the specific things you absolutely hate. Just because running burns the most calories and you're trying to lose weight doesn't mean you should take up running if you know you hate it. Don't let friends, family members, social trends, or even your personal trainer decide which type of exercise is right for you. The best type of exercise is the one that you will do consistently, day after day, and week after week.

In order to find one or two things you don't totally hate, you'll have to try new things. If you've never tried jogging, don't assume you'll hate it. There are plenty of activities you can work into your exercise program, so don't limit yourself to the usual suspects (cardio machines, weight lifting, cardio classes). Take this opportunity to go beyond your normal comfort zone. You're making personality changes with the goal of improving your physical self, but you can use those physical activities as an opportunity to make personality improvements too! Get creative with this and try every new activity at least twice before you decide you don't like it. Try speed walking, spinning, Frisbee golf, Krav Maga, Latin dance, qigong—there is almost no limit to the number of activities you can do, and there are tons of resources you can seek out to spark new ideas.

The final tip I have for you right now is to start off slowly and not be overly ambitious. I'll get into why later on, but for now just trust that it is important.

## ✐ Exercise 16: Overcome Your Inertia.

This exercise is pretty simple. You will decide how often and for how long you will exercise for the coming week and then keep track of how well you do by adding a journal entry in your notebook (not on your food log). For now, don't worry about counting how many calories you're burning, unless you find that motivational and you want to. Your focus with this exercise is to start forming the habit of doing some type of planned physical activity *every* day, or at least on most days of the week. I know that sounds ridiculous if you haven't been exercising at all, but I'll tell you why it's better to exercise for a short time every day than it is to exercise longer only a few times per week: habit. Exercising every day is a very strong habit that's hard to break once it's taken root, whereas exercising two or three times a week is barely a habit at all. When you're not exercising daily, it's far too easy to say, "Well, I didn't get to my workout today, but I can make it up tomorrow." Soon your three workouts a week become two, and from there exercise becomes something sporadic rather than something habitual.

The good news is, you don't have to exercise for very long when you're just starting out. In fact, I urge you to set *very realistic* goals for the amount of time you want to spend being active each day, and entirely ignore accomplishments in terms of calories burned, miles traveled, pounds lifted, etc. For this exercise, your focus should be only on forming the habit of exercise. Also, at least for the first few weeks, your effort level should only be light to moderate and not vigorous at all.

Depending on your current physical condition and your schedule, you may need to spread your active minutes across two or three different bouts during the day. Say you've decided to start with a goal of 15 minutes of activity every day for the first two weeks. If you're obese, suffer from a chronic condition, are severely out of shape, or have other physically limiting factors at play, it may not be *safe* for you to sustain even light activity for 15 continuous minutes. (Everyone embarking on an exercise program for the first time, or after a long sedentary period, should consult with a physician before beginning such a program.) Or perhaps you really can't carve out a 15-minute chunk of time on one or two days of the week when your schedule is particularly hectic. In this case you might need to do a 10-minute bout and a 5-minute bout, or three 5-minute bouts, on a particular day.

In this first phase, no amount of time is too small—really! The important thing is to get into the habit of preplanning your exercise at the beginning of each week, and then making sure you stick to your plan.

Before I give you the character example for this exercise, let me tell you the story of one of my clients who was overly ambitious. This gentleman swore to me the first day we met that he was going to exercise 40 minutes a day, five days a week after having done nothing at all for years. I urged him to start smaller, maybe 10 or 15 minutes a day, but no, if he was going to do this, then he was going to do it right! Except he never did it. He could never carve out 40 minutes in a day, and so he *never* exercised except the one day each week when I showed up for our session. Needless to say, he was not one of my success stories. Even if you are more dedicated and motivated than he was, I still urge you to take it easy in the beginning. There's a tendency to get excited about this new endeavor and go "all out." I call this the honeymoon phase, and it usually lasts about three weeks, but it can quickly lead to burnout or, in worse cases, injury. Instead, I recommend you follow Bob's example.

## Character Example

Bob strongly dislikes exercise. He doesn't think he'll ever get to the point where he considers it something he wants to do, so he knows he'll need to think of it as something he has to do. Here's what he writes in his notebook:

*Exercise 16: Overcome My Inertia.*

*I hate to exercise, but I have to do it. Starting today, I will exercise for at least 15 minutes every day this week. I'll mostly stick to walking, because I don't know if I'm able to do much else, but tomorrow I'll check out the fitness room at work and see what I think I can add. Today I'll go for a walk outside right after I'm done with this journal entry, and I'll put the rest of my planned workouts on my calendar, with alerts turned on so that I don't forget. I'll need to remember to bring a change of clothes if I'm going to exercise at work. More on that tomorrow.*

Bob opens his calendar, scans each day, and finds a place to fit exercise in for at least 15 minutes. Then he closes his calendar and changes into sweatpants and sneakers and heads out the door for his first walk. He starts off at a brisk pace, excited about this new commitment, but he's surprised at how quickly he becomes tired. He remembers that he's supposed to be keeping his effort light or moderate, so he slows down and spends the rest of his walk intentionally enjoying his surroundings.

## Why You Should Keep Exercise Out of Your Food Log

You might be wondering why I'm not letting you track your exercise on your food log when there's probably a handy place for you to enter it there. The reason why will come into play once you actually start tracking calories daily, and it has to do with our old nemesis, inaccuracy. It also happens to be a big reason why so many people fail to lose weight through exercise alone.

Do you remember the calorie-counting trap I described in the last chapter—the story about the woman who was scrimping and saving her calories all day long so that she could "spend" them on junk food or booze in the evening? Well, there's a similar calorie-counting trap people often fall into with exercise.

Imagine another kind of calorie "saver"—one who carefully records everything he eats all day long and consistently comes to find that he's going to have to eat a measly dinner in order to hit his calorie target for the day. "Ah, I know!" he thinks. "I'll just exercise and burn a few hundred calories so I can eat more for dinner." The trouble is, this gentleman is like most people in that he will routinely underestimate his calories consumed (for reasons previously discussed) and overestimate his calories burned.

In the case of calories burned, the error is partly due to the very generic formulas most programs or calculators use to guess at your very unique basal metabolic rate (BMR), which represents how many calories you burn per minute if you are doing nothing at all. There are so many factors that contribute to a person's BMR that it would be impossible for a basic computer program to get it right. So what you get instead is a reasonable estimate, which can be off by a significant amount.

A further problem with estimating calories burned is the difference between net calories and gross calories. Gross calories burned through activity is the total number of calories your body burned while you were exercising. So, say our man here walks briskly for 30 minutes and burns 200 calories. He plugs that into his food log and it "gives" him 200 extra calories to eat for dinner. Great! Oh, except that if he had been sitting on the couch during those 30 minutes, he still would have burned about 45 to 60 calories (depending on his individual metabolic factors). So to be accurate, he should have only allowed himself around 150 extra calories. A difference of 50 calories may not seem like much, but when added up over the course of a month, it becomes more significant.[8]

Now consider the even worse case—that this gentleman may actually be getting credit for his exercise calories *twice*. Remember the step in Exercise 15 where you entered your activity level into your food log settings? Most people tend to report that they are "somewhat active" or "active" depending on how many times per week they exercise because that's what many programs use to gauge activity level. So let's say our guy told his program that he is "somewhat active" because he typically exercises three times per week. The program then calculates his daily calorie allowance *based on the fact that he has already reported a higher level of activity* regardless of whether he actually does exercise three times per week or not. Each day this man is told that he can consume 50 or 100 more calories than he would have if he'd reported that, in fact, he is sedentary because he sits at a desk all day, sits in a car on his way to work and back home, and spends most of the evening sitting on the sofa. So on those days when he does exercise, he is merely meeting the criteria he already told the calorie calculator to factor in for him, and he should get no credit for these exercise calories unless they go above and beyond the level of activity he reported (a difficult thing to determine).

Certain food log programs or apps and a few websites with calculators that estimate BMR will correctly use activity exclusive of exercise to determine which category a person falls into. They may also calculate net, rather than gross, calories expended. The program used in Cindy's Exercise 15 is one such example. However, I have found that in all cases, once you start tracking daily calorie totals, *not* entering exercise into the food log equation will yield better weight-loss results. This is why I strongly encourage you to track your activity separately and not fall into this particular calorie-counting trap. It's a great idea, in fact, to track and report your exercise in a public forum, like on your social media account, via e-mail or text message to your trainer, or to your virtual or in-person weight-loss group. This holds you accountable and keeps you motivated in a much more positive way than simply exercising so that you can eat a little bit more that day.

# Chapter Six

# SET YOURSELF UP FOR SUCCESS

In the preceding two chapters, you picked the first few dietary behaviors you want to modify, and you committed to exercising daily. Depending on which behaviors you chose to target and on how resistant you're feeling about the exercise thing, you might be feeling pretty confident and excited right now, or you might be getting that sinking feeling that this is already too difficult. If you're feeling confident and excited, then celebrate that! Pay attention to what this feels like and store it away, because sooner or later, you'll come up against a challenge that will leave you feeling unsure about your abilities to stick with the program. If you're feeling that way right now, then I'd like to give you some strategies you can use to build your confidence and regain positive motivation.

First, think about why you're feeling the way you are. Are your feelings fear based? Do they have some foundation in your past attempts and failures to lose weight? If that's the case, then you should go back in your notebook to Exercises 3 and 4. Reread your positive self-talk statements and take yourself through your positive visualization exercises again. Remember that things are different this time; you're making different commitments and applying new knowledge and strategies to an old problem. You are a different person now—a fit, thin person, perhaps not in body yet, but in mind. Observe your fears and, without judging, know that they are just that. Your fears are something you will have to deal with, but they are not a part of you unless you let them be.

Next, ask yourself whether you might have chosen a behavior or two that were a little too ambitious for this stage of the game. If you targeted the things that would have the biggest impact, and if those things are proving very difficult for you to change, then maybe you'll have to redo Exercise 14 and go for the "low-hanging fruit" instead and choose one or two behaviors that are the easiest for you to change. They might not result in the biggest bang for your calorie-cutting buck, but the upside is that you gain valuable practice at working through the behavior change process and success is highly probable. Remember that early success builds confidence and motivation. This approach can help you be more successful later, when it's time to face those more difficult behaviors.

 ## Exercise 17: Reassess Your Motivation and Your Plan.

Before moving on to Step 9, take a few moments and write down where you are emotionally with everything right now. If you need to, go back and redo Exercises 3 and 4, and/or Exercise 14. When you're feeling reasonably confident about everything, move on to the next step. We'll skip the character example for this exercise—you've got this one!

## Step Nine:
# IDENTIFY YOUR BARRIERS TO CHANGE

In order to be successful this time around, it's important to identify all of the little reasons why your unhealthy habits existed in the first place. If behavior change was easy, you wouldn't need to make an effort to lose weight at all, would you? You'd just change the stuff you know is responsible for your weight gain. But behavior change is not easy because there are so many barriers out there.

A barrier to change is anything that can jump out and block your progress while you're diligently trying to alter your behaviors. Here's an example: Say one of your first key behaviors is "I eat too many empty calories at work. I will start bringing healthier snacks to work and say no when someone offers me junk food." When trying to change that behavior, what's likely to get in your way? Boredom; coworkers who bring in baked goods; unhealthy food brought by management to staff meetings; junk food in the vending machines; your failure to bring a healthy lunch and snacks . . . the list goes on. Each one of these things is a possible barrier to changing the habit of "eating too many empty calories at work." In this step you'll identify your own barriers for each of the behaviors you've decided to tackle first.

If you've been working on those behaviors for a few days, then you may have noticed some barriers already. In addition to those, I also want you to think about your past efforts to lose weight and brainstorm an extensive list of previous barriers. It's important to take this step, because knowing what difficulties you might run into ahead of time makes it easier for you to work through them when they arise, and you'll be more likely to stick with your new healthy habits.

## ✐ Exercise 18: For Each of Your Dietary and Exercise Behaviors, List All Possible Barriers.

This exercise is straight-forward, but might be a little time-consuming. Brainstorm every possible thing that could creep up and set you back. Be exhaustive here, looking at both internal and external barriers. Name all the conditions or situations that are likely to hinder your progress. There's no barrier too small to be included: special occasions, work and social gatherings, an upcoming vacation, your daily commute past a favorite restaurant, the ritual morning coffee break with coworkers, Pizza Fridays, generous coworkers who bring in treats, lack of time to exercise, dislike of exercise, potential illnesses or injuries, unsupportive family members or friends—you get the idea. Also be as *specific* as possible: which restaurants, which foods exactly, name the names of people who might be a hindrance, what forms of exercise you absolutely hate, which part of your body you have injured in the past, which illnesses you are prone to getting. Think of every last possible tiny little hindrance you can imagine.

It can be helpful to write out your barriers as sentences that show a specific cause-effect relationship: "When _____, I tend to _____." Example: "When I don't get enough sleep, I tend to get coffee and a high-calorie snack mid-morning, and skip my workout later in the day," or "When I visit my friend Julie, I tend to drink a lot more wine than when I'm on my own or with other friends." Whatever you've put in the first blank is a barrier to changing the behavior in the second blank.

# Character Example

In Exercise 14, Bob decided that his first two dietary behaviors would be to eat breakfast at home every morning and to eat an apple and take a short walk when he was feeling stressed rather than to eat something unhealthy or drink alcohol. You'll recall that in Exercise 16, he committed to 15 minutes of exercise every day. Here is his list of barriers for those habits:

*Exercise 18: List All Possible Barriers to Change.*

1. *I will eat a healthy breakfast at home every morning.*

    *Time: I have a bad habit of snoozing through my alarm and running late in the morning. When I wake up late, I skip breakfast at home and eat something less healthy on the way to work.*

    *Lack of options: We mostly just have kids' cereal and sugary instant oatmeal in the house. When there's nothing for me to eat at home, I skip breakfast and eat something on the way to work.*

    *Temptation: I drive right by the BigBop every morning, and I love their breakfast croissant sandwiches. When I see the BigBop, I often give in to the temptation to stop and get a croissant sandwich.*

2. *When I am feeling stressed out, I will go for a five-minute walk and eat an apple instead of eating junk food or drinking alcohol.*

    *Habit: It's second nature for me to reach for my usual "comfort" foods or drinks. It's going to be hard to remember not to do this and to substitute the healthy behaviors instead. When I'm not mindful of my eating and drinking behaviors, I automatically make poor choices.*

    *Ability: I often feel stressed at work when things are busy. I may not be able to take five minutes to go for a walk right then. Often my stress eating occurs on my way home from work or when I get home. When I don't take time to relax during the day, I let loose once I get home, "rewarding" myself with bad food or alcohol.*

    *Apples: I'll have to buy lots of them and keep them on hand. When I don't have a healthy alternative readily available, I automatically turn to my comfort foods.*

    *Beer/Other Alcohol: After a long, stressful day, I usually go for a beer right away. One usually turns into two or three. It's a habit as automatic as breathing. When I'm stressed and tired, I am not mindful of my drinking behaviors. On some level I think this is a bit intentional. I ignore the truth because I tell myself that having alcohol feels good.*

3. *I will exercise for at least 15 minutes every day.*

*Attitude: I hate to exercise. I'm afraid I'll look for excuses to avoid it. When I am faced with doing something I dislike, I make excuses for not doing it.*

*Time: I know 15 minutes isn't much, but I'm worried this will be one of the main excuses I try to use. When I don't prioritize exercise in my daily schedule, I tend to skip it.*

*Weather: I'll be walking outside after work most of the time, so I can see using bad weather as an excuse. When it's very cold outside, I am likely to skip my walk outdoors.*

*Shyness/Embarrassment: I could exercise at work, but I feel intimidated and embarrassed because I'm so fat. When I let my fear of embarrassment get to me, I let it dictate my actions.*

*Clothing: I only have one pair of sweatpants and a couple of T-shirts that I can fit into, and they're in pretty rough shape. I'd be embarrassed to be seen wearing them at work. Again, when I let my fear of embarrassment get to me, I let it dictate my actions.*

## A Brief Discussion About Barriers

Before we move on to the next step, I want to address the issue of barriers and to stress the importance of being able to recognize and counteract them.

Remember those grim statistics about weight-loss success rates—only 20 percent of those who lose weight will keep it off. There are a few common reasons (barriers) why so many people fail, and if you know what they are, keep an eye out for them throughout your process, and have a plan in place for how to deal with them when they pop up, you'll have a greater chance for success.

First off, many people lose pretty large amounts of weight over relatively short periods of time by engaging in fairly extreme diet and exercise programs. This type of dieting is actually a causal factor for weight *gain*,[1] and the underlying barriers associated with it are impatience (the desire or expectation to lose weight more quickly than is rational) and unrealistic expectations in the goal-setting step. If you need to drop a quick 15 or 20 pounds for a special occasion and do not care to achieve permanent weight loss, then these kinds of diets can be effective—*but only if you do so once or twice in your whole life!* "Weight-cycling," or the repeated pattern of losing and then regaining weight, is potentially dangerous[2] and has been associated with higher BMI and abdominal fat accumulation.[3] Thinking that you'll drop a quick 20 pounds on a crash diet and then sustain that weight loss by employing more sound habits is a recipe for disaster. Fortunately, in this process you have formulated realistic goals, committing to long-term lifestyle change, which does not include fad diet and exercise programs, so you don't have to worry about this. Just be aware that there is a lot of marketing out there that will try to convince you otherwise. Remember that these corporations are trying to sell you something—they have their own bottom line, and not your best interest, in mind. Don't get sucked in by the promise of fantastic results. Stick with your program, even if progress is slower than you prefer.

Another big reason why people regain their weight is stress. There are different kinds of stress, though. There is the stress of daily life, which we all experience in varying quantities. This kind of stress can often be controlled to some degree by the choices you make, and your reaction to this stress is often more important than the stressors themselves. Everyday stress should not be used as an excuse for lack of progress—it is an obstacle that you can fairly easily overcome.

But what about that other kind of stress—the kind that comes with major life events like the death of a loved one, your own or another family member's diagnosis with a serious disease, the loss or change of your job, moving to a new area where you don't know anyone, etc. These types of events can spark strong and deep-seated emotional coping mechanisms, which can result in behaviors like emotional eating, abuse of alcohol, and other causal factors for weight gain. Also, depression often accompanies these stressful events, and a person's energy can be sapped, reducing the amount of effort they are willing to devote to exercise, grocery shopping, and preparation of healthy food. In other words, those healthy habits you just spent months forming can fall by the wayside quickly when you are consumed by a life-altering event. It is understandable, to be sure.

While this type of obstacle is rare and very difficult to overcome, there are a few things you can do to help mitigate the effects it can have on your goals. The most important of these is to seek help in managing your stress and depression. When serious stress events envelope your life, the most important thing you can do is to seek professional guidance. Now is not the time to be tough and go it alone.

The one thing you can do on your own, however, is use logic to propel yourself forward when you'd rather curl up in a ball and quit participating in life. It is well-known that exercise relieves symptoms of depression and boosts energy levels and immune function, providing yet another reason for you to continue exercising in the midst of your crisis. Also, in situations like this, it often feels like you have control over nothing in your life, but you do, in fact, have control over your own body, what you feed it, and what kinds of activities you do. For those who are thrust into a battle with cancer or who have suffered a heart attack, the type and intensity of physical activity will certainly change, but returning to light activity as soon as possible can be one of the best therapies. If you find that you're suddenly forced to care for a loved one and think you no longer have time to keep up your new habits, remember that you are only as good to others as you are to yourself. Neglecting your own needs will wear you down and possibly cultivate resentment toward the very person you are trying to be there for. So take care of yourself first, and then take care of everyone else who depends on you.

Finally, there are some barriers that people may never recognize because they lie beneath the surface, deeply imbedded within them. These barriers are those larger emotional reasons that have caused an endless cycle of weight gain over years or decades. People who struggle with these kinds of issues want to believe that if they simply change their behaviors, the pounds will come off and stay off for good. But they're ignoring the fact that *behaviors can only truly change when the mind changes.* If the underlying mental and emotional reasons that have led to weight-gain behaviors are not removed, then it's only a matter of time before the new, healthy behaviors start to erode. So it's most important to look within yourself as you compile your list of barriers. Ask yourself what feelings, attitudes, fears, and assumptions you are bringing to this process that might be counterproductive. Be aware that years of thinking and feeling certain ways about food, stress, rest, and exercise have created negative lifestyle habits and have added pounds that will come off much more stubbornly than they went on. Unless you change the *why* involved, the *what* is not likely to matter much over the long term.

## 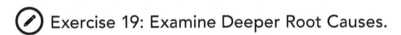 Exercise 19: Examine Deeper Root Causes.

Identifying those day-to-day behaviors you engage in that contribute to your poor condition is important, but it's not the only thing that matters. In order to get to your real "why," you will need to deeply examine the internal picture by looking at your whole, long history and identifying the key factors *within you* that have led to where you are today. This is not an exercise that can be accomplished by filling out a questionnaire or making a simple list. Rather, you should keep a detailed and ongoing journal, recounting events and memories from your past as well as current events in your life, feelings, etc. This is a process that might go on for months. You probably won't have an "aha!" moment that provides you with instant insight; rather, it will be a slow process of discovery. You don't have to finish this exercise entirely before moving on to the next steps, but you should spend some time with it now, exploring the true root causes of your weight gain. Seeing a therapist might be time and money well spent if you can afford it. Ignoring this exercise and pressing right on to more difficult behavior changes is not very likely to deliver the results you are looking for.

## Character Example

Bob isn't looking forward to this exercise. He knows there are a lot of "demons" in his past, from the way his eating habits differed from other kids' when he was young, to turning to food for comfort whenever he was upset as a child, to the many crazy beer and pizza frat parties in college that grew his capacity to eat and drink exponentially. He buys a separate small notebook for this exercise so that he can continue to write in it as he simultaneously works through the rest of the steps. For several days, he focuses mightily on this exercise, writing in detail about everything he can think of that has contributed to his unhealthy habits on a deeper level. Much of it is hard to think about and write down, but as he does, answers begin to emerge to some of the questions he's had about why it's been so hard for him to lose weight and keep it off. There are a few things that jump out at him as recurring themes, and he knows he'll need to watch out for them as he moves forward this time around.

## Step Ten:

# CLASSIFY YOUR BARRIERS AND PRACTICE DEFEATING THEM

When you consider all the internal barriers along with all the external pressures and temptations to eat poorly and to be sedentary, you might wonder how anyone has ever lost any weight at all! But take comfort in the fact that many, many people have done just that. Twenty percent of millions is a huge number, and what has differentiated that successful 20 percent, perhaps more than anything else, is *their ability to overcome the obstacles they encountered while keeping focused on their goals.*

The bad news is that there is no magic secret for how to lose weight. The good news is that there is no magic secret for how to lose weight! You do it the same way you accomplish any task you set out to do—methodically, strategically, and persistently.

## Formulate Your Plan of Attack

Think about a work or school project you have recently completed. What process did you use to get it done? If it was a big undertaking, you may have looked at it before you started and thought, "How am I supposed to do this?" But you laid out a plan, you broke it down into manageable pieces, and you rolled up your sleeves and got to work. You worked persistently, dealing with problems as they popped up, and you dealt with your frustration rather than giving up when things became difficult. Things didn't go perfectly for you; you had to adapt and be creative. You kept on working until the project was completed. Weight loss is just like that. It's a project that you need to work on, and once you've decided that you *need* to work on it and *will* finish it, then the only thing standing in your way are those obstacles that will inevitably arise. If you are able to learn how to manage and overcome those barriers, your success is all but guaranteed. The next two exercises will help you do that.

The first exercise will ask you to classify your barriers into one of three categories: those you can avoid, those you'll have to get around, and those you'll have to tackle head-on. Let's take a look at these three categories.

### *Barriers That Can Be Avoided*

There will be many barriers to change that you can eliminate simply by altering your environment so that you're never faced with them in the first place. These obstacles are normally encountered under specific circumstances or in specific locations that you have some control over. For example, let's say you know that when you're running short on time and you drive past a favorite restaurant on your way home from work, you frequently stop and grab a quick burger and fries because it's convenient and you love their food. There are two barriers here: one is the restaurant, and the other is your love of their fattening food. Changing your love for that kind of food is hard, but avoiding that particular restaurant is pretty easy—you can simply drive home along a different route that doesn't take you past that restaurant, right?

Another example of an avoidable barrier is that friend of yours who only wants to get together with you if it involves happy hour drinks and appetizers at her favorite restaurant. There are a few barriers in this case: your friend, the activity that you and she do together (going out to happy hour), your inability to say no to her invitations, and your inability to say no to the appetizer platter. If she's a close friend, then of course you want to continue your relationship with her, so that's probably not a barrier you want to eliminate. If you get good at saying no to her invitations, she might eliminate you as a friend—also undesirable. But what if you could still hang out with your friend and simply avoid happy hour? That would be okay, wouldn't it? To do this, you'll have to sit down with her and have a heart-to-heart. You'll have to come up with some alternative activity the two of you can do, and in that way, you'll be able to avoid the situations you find so difficult. If your friend isn't on board with this, then perhaps she actually *is* the obstacle you need to eliminate. You'll need to decide whether she's worth compromising your goals for.

The fact that you can avoid some barriers doesn't necessarily make them easy to defeat, but avoiding a barrier is the surest way of overcoming it, so given the choice, it's always best to try to do so.

### *Barriers That Can Be Circumnavigated*

Sometimes you can't avoid the situations where barriers lurk. The workplace comes to mind here, as does the concession stand at your daughter's basketball game. You have to be in that place at that time, and the tempting food is there. It's not practical for you to leave, but it is possible for you to "get around" the barriers in these situations. In the workplace, for example, the best way to keep from being tempted by all of the goodies coworkers bring in is to let them know that you don't want any of it . . . ever. When coworkers offer you a sweet treat or a slice of pizza, politely tell them that you're in the process of losing weight and getting healthy and those things are not part of the program. Thank them for offering and then tell them that it would be helpful to you if they just didn't offer similar things to you in the future. Then be sure to avoid those areas where the tempting treats tend to gather. One of my clients actually posted a sign at her cubicle reminding her well-meaning coworkers not to offer treats to her: "Thanks, but no thanks—Linda is on a diet!" was written below a cartoon drawing of a cupcake. The tempting food was still there, but Linda wasn't exposed to it nearly as often.

Circumnavigating a barrier is the next best thing to not having to encounter it at all. Look for ways that you can alter your routine, your route of travel, or your interaction with certain people so that even though the obstacle is nearby, you're not forced to confront it directly.

*Barriers That Must Be Defeated Using Willpower*

Finally, there are some situations over which you really have no control. You're stuck in a staff meeting with your boss and there's a box full of donuts in the center of the table. You're at a holiday party and there are trays full of delicacies and drinks being offered around. It's your son's fifth birthday party and you have to buy or bake him a cake.

In these situations, there is nothing you can do to remove yourself from the obstacle, and you can't distance yourself from it, so you're forced to defeat it using sheer willpower. This is very difficult to do, and should be avoided if at all possible. There are some things you can do that will help you get through those tough moments. We'll get to those right after you complete this next exercise.

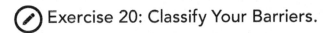 Exercise 20: Classify Your Barriers.

Look at your list of barriers from Exercise 18. Think about the circumstances in which you're likely to encounter each of them, and then categorize each one as Avoid, Circumnavigate, or Defeat. Then for each one jot down some strategies or steps you'll have to implement in order to successfully do so.

## Character Example

Taking the lists of barriers Bob made for each of his key behaviors in Example 18, he works to put them into three categories: Avoid, Circumnavigate, and Defeat. Here is how Bob's barriers break down:

*Avoid:*
- *BigBop Temptation: I can take a different route home. Taking Shepherd Avenue will get me home in about the same amount of time, and there are no restaurants along that route that I'll be tempted to stop at.*
- *Stress Drinking (Beer/Alcohol): I will have to stop buying booze. I'm the only one who drinks it at home, so it won't be hard just to not have it around. I like sparkling water well enough, so I'll try using that as a substitute with meals where I would normally have a beer. I'll have to address drinking beer and cocktails when I'm out with friends, colleagues, and clients in the defeat category as well.*

- *Shyness/Embarrassment of Exercising at Work: At least in the beginning, I think I should try to exercise at home as much as possible. Once I've built up a little confidence, maybe I can try to defeat this barrier by overcoming my insecurities, but I don't think that's realistic right now.*

*Circumnavigate:*

- *No Time for Breakfast: I will set two alarms every night and put one on the dresser across the room. I'll also tell my wife not to let me back into bed after my alarms go off in the morning.*
- *Lack of Breakfast Options at Home: I'll get some healthier cereals, keep eggs and whole-grain bread on hand, and start setting the coffeemaker the night before so my coffee is ready to go each morning. This will encourage me to sit down and eat before I start my hectic day.*
- *Forgetting/Lack of Mindfulness: I will make lists of my key behaviors and post them on my desk, my office door, in my car, and anyplace else where I'll be sure to see them. To get in the habit of going for a walk at work, I'll initially set an alarm for every hour and take a short walk break down the hall and back as often as I am able. I'll tell my coworkers and boss about this new habit so that they can be supportive.*
- *Apples vs. Junk Food: Obviously I'll need to buy some apples! I'll bring a small bag to the office every Monday and keep another bag at home. I'll use the bathroom at the other end of the building so I don't have to pass by the break room and the vending machines. I'll let my coworkers know that if they ever see me standing at the vending machine, they should ask me if I've run out of apples. I'll tell my wife and son to do the same at home when they see me scanning the refrigerator contents for a snack.*
- *No Time to Exercise: I will exercise first thing when I get home every evening, before I'm allowed to eat dinner. If I'm meeting clients out in the evening, I will exercise that morning— I'll set my two alarms 20 minutes earlier than usual.*

*Defeat:*

- *Alcohol in Social or Work Situations: I know this is a big threat to my progress because I am out with clients or colleagues several nights a week. I'm often uncomfortable in these situations because of my weight, so I drink to "loosen up." I'll need to learn how to manage my stress and stick to water or sparkling water in these situations. I can recruit my coworker, Jim, to help me—we are pretty good friends, and he almost always attends the same events I do. I might get some pressure from a few of the guys at the firm, but I'll let them know that it's part of my weight-loss program, and they should understand. Telling them about it will also add another layer of accountability and discourage me from drinking when I'm in their company. Football Sundays at Mom's house is another situation I'll have to address in a similar way, and my brother probably won't be an ally. He likes to drink, and he likes to have company. If it becomes too much to deal with, I'll have to stop going to Mom's to watch the game, but I hope it doesn't come to that.*

- *Bad Attitude Toward Exercise: I'll make a list of all those great benefits of exercise and staple a copy of the picture of me in my senior yearbook onto the margin. I'll hang a copy up on my office door and on the bathroom mirror. I know if I can keep my motivation high, I can overcome this barrier. I used to love working out in college. I just need to get over these tough first few weeks.*

## Tips for Defeating Unavoidable Barriers

The most important thing you can do—if you remember nothing else, remember this—is to *stay focused on your goal and take your focus off of the barrier.* By shifting your thinking immediately to your goal—your very specific, well-defined goal—you bolster your willpower exponentially. Immediately and in the forefront of your mind, you will have the motivation and the reason why you're trying to resist this temptation and overcome this barrier. Next, you want to *divert your attention away from the barrier* as quickly as possible. Don't look at it; don't think about it; don't talk about it.

In social and familial situations, others may try to focus your attention directly on the barrier. They will offer it to you dozens of times; they will waft its scrumptious aroma into your face; they will *ooh* and *ahh* and tell you how wonderful it is and how much you're missing out. I could make the argument that these people are not really your friends, but that's for you to decide. What I will suggest is that you take that opportunity, right then, to communicate sincerely and effectively with them. Without getting emotional or angry, tell them that you have a goal you're working very hard to achieve, they are presently acting as an obstacle to that goal, and you would appreciate very much if they would support you in your efforts rather than create setbacks for you. And then see how they react. Your part is done, and the only thing you have left to do is decide if this is something you want to expose yourself to in the future.

In situations where other people are not the barrier, but something more seemingly "fixed" is, such as a lack of time to exercise, an unexpected injury, etc., you'll have to think creatively in order to overcome it.

There will be days when you run short on time. Seemingly catastrophic things will happen to your schedule that will make it seem impossible to get in a workout. On days like this, it is very important to give no ground to your obstacles. The best way to defeat a barrier like this is to *plan ahead*. In this case, a lack of time for exercise requires a solution that is preplanned and quick to implement. Having your workout clothes packed in a bag and always with you is one way you can be ready to exercise at a moment's notice. At the very least, having a pair of shoes and a T-shirt you can change into for a brisk walk is a necessity. You'll also want to have a short, higher-intensity workout in your repertoire for times when 10 or 15 minutes is all you can spare. There are a number of these workouts published on reputable fitness websites, or you can get one from your trainer. It's important to have tried this workout ahead of time so that you're familiar with it. Learning something new and trying it for the first time when you're in a rush is a bad idea. Finally, you may just need to get creative. If you don't have 15 minutes, if you're already late to pick up the kids and get them to school in time for their band concert, then you'll need to improvise. Get your kids, get to the school, drop them off where they need to be, and tell them you're going to park the car. Then go walk around the block for 15 minutes. Trust me, the remaining 45 minutes of off-key band music will be more than you want to hear anyway.

The *key* element to all of this, though, is that *you must PRACTICE defeating barriers.* Practice having that conversation with your friends at the restaurant before you leave home. Practice politely turning down dessert from your aunt all eight times she will offer it to you. Practice your short, hard exercise routine, and practice walking in your business skirt, tennis shoes, and T-shirt in the middle of the day sometime when you are not in a rush (that way you'll know if you need to keep a towel and deodorant in your desk drawer).

*When things are going wrong, that's not the time to add more stress to the situation by trying something new.*

That's the time to pull out the tools you've already practiced. They will be a comfort to you, giving you back some measure of control over a situation that would otherwise be both frustrating and damaging to your goals.

Practicing ahead of time also gives you the opportunity to fail when it doesn't matter. Finding out that a strategy doesn't work when you're in the middle of an uncontrolled situation can be very damaging to your motivation. But finding that out when you're exploring possibilities is a positive learning tool that allows you to go back to the drawing board and come up with another, more effective strategy.

##  Exercise 21: Practice Defeating Unavoidable Barriers.

Look at the barriers you've put in the Defeat category. For each one, write a detailed script outlining the exact steps you'll take to overcome them when they arise. But don't stop there! Having something on paper is a good start, but to really be successful, you need to have practice and hands-on experience implementing your strategies. The more specific you can be to each situation and the more realistic you can make your practice sessions, the better. Get one of your trusted allies to play the role of a pushy friend as you come up with your planned responses to their cajoling. Have your role-playing partner be tough on you too. Even have some tempting food around that you can practice rejecting in a safe environment. It will build your confidence and make it a lot easier when you're out there in the shark tank.

## Character Example

Cindy asks her friend Mark to play the role of Cindy's best friend, Sherry. Cindy and Sherry meet for happy hour nearly every Friday, and sometimes on other days of the week too. When Cindy told everyone about her weight-loss goals back in Exercise 5, Sherry was less than thrilled. Since then, Sherry has been putting on the pressure to get Cindy out for drinks and bar food. To make the exercise as realistic as possible, Cindy and Mark go out to the restaurant Cindy and Sherry most frequently go to, and they go during happy hour.

Cindy has done her homework ahead of time, looking at the menu online and selecting those food items that fall within her current eating plan. She has also set a rule for herself—she'll have one glass of wine and then switch to water after that. This too falls in line with her dietary goals.

Cindy asks Mark to pretend to be Sherry and to be hard on her. Mark relentlessly tries to get Cindy to split the appetizer platter with him. He orders a frozen margarita—one of Cindy's favorite drinks (which contains far more calories than her glass of wine does)—and he keeps offering sips of it to her. Halfway through the evening, he even pretends to break out of his role and tries to convince Cindy to indulge a little with him: "You can have one more glass of wine here with me, can't you? You wouldn't be busting your weekly limit, right?" But Cindy stands firm, and when she does, Mark congratulates her. Cindy feels ready for the real thing with Sherry now.

Know that defeating obstacles will almost never be easy. We develop habits primarily out of laziness (or "efficiency," to put it more politely) and/or for instant gratification. We want to get there faster, using as little energy as possible; we want to eat that thing that tastes so good right now, disregarding the long-term effects that it will have. This is the tough work you'll need to do in order to lose weight and keep it off. It's a good idea to recall your reasons for wanting to lose weight, and your positive visualization, frequently. When motivation is high, success comes rather easily, but if you lose sight of your goal and your reasons for setting that goal, then obstacles quickly become excuses and you end up not sticking with your efforts. If you let that continue for more than a day or two, then suddenly your whole effort is in jeopardy. Imagine where you'd be in life if you carried that attitude and type of behavior into your professional work! You would generally be a pretty unsuccessful person. But you are *not* that way in other areas of your life, and so you can draw from those skill sets and apply those positive habits to this effort as well. You *can* find ways to avoid or work around your obstacles to weight loss, and if you are to be successful, you must!

## Chapter Seven

# STEP IT UP A NOTCH

Ihope you've had a successful first week or two of getting in *some* exercise every day. If you haven't, then read the section on Frequency below and spend another week or two working to lay a solid foundation for daily exercise.

Once you have been exercising regularly, it's time to start getting more out of your workouts, both in terms of calories burned and health-boosting benefits. There are a few ways you can do that, but right now you should only choose one of them. I'll give you a synopsis of the different aspects of exercise, and then it will be up to you to choose which one you'll focus on right now.

## Step Eleven:
## GET MORE FROM YOUR WORKOUTS

### Getting FIT

There's a handy acronym that describes the variables that go into a workout: *FIT*—Frequency, *Intensity, Time*. Sometimes you might see another *T* tacked on at the end, and this stands for "Type," which I'll talk about a little bit later. For now I don't want to throw too many new things at you, so if you've found one or two activities that you enjoy well enough to do every day, let's stick with those for a while.

## Frequency: When More Matters Most

I've already been harping on this, so it shouldn't surprise you to learn that I think frequency is the most important component of exercise. One major reason for this is that many of the wonderful health benefits of exercise are very short-lived, but if you exercise daily, you can enjoy those benefits all the time. For example, the mood-boosting and blood pressure–lowering effects of exercise last for a few hours after a workout, so if you suffer from depression, anxiety, chronic stress, or hypertension, then daily exercise can be a highly effective treatment for these conditions.[1] If you only exercise three or four days per week, then you'll get those benefits only on those days, and the cumulative effect of your sessions might not be enough to make more permanent metabolic changes (lowering your blood pressure all the time, for example). That's one reason why frequency is the most important variable to focus on when you're just starting out. The other reason we've already discussed—doing something every day quickly builds those neural pathways that result in forming a positive habit.[2]

If you haven't been active every day up to now, then your primary exercise-related goal is forming that habit. A good strategy is to add one extra day per week to what you've been able to do so far. So, if up to now you've been getting in a 15-minute workout three days per week, next week you should aim for four days, and so on. Eventually you should aim to do something *every day*, but you can consider yourself successful if at the end of a month you have completed twenty-seven or twenty-eight workouts.

## Time: Keep Your Eye on the Clock

Time is the next variable I'll address. In this case, "time" doesn't refer to the time of day, but rather the duration of your exercise bouts. Once you're working out daily, your total weekly calorie expenditure from exercise will result from some product of time and intensity. If you have been sedentary for a long time and are generally unfit, then you will *have* to address time before intensity. It simply isn't safe for a deconditioned individual to work out harder until their level of fitness has increased substantially, and increasing the duration of your workouts will help you do this.

In Exercise 16 you established your baseline workout duration based on how much time you were willing to set aside for exercise and your current level of fitness. In this next phase, to increase the time variable you should set miniature weekly goals to increase the duration of your exercise sessions. Think really small here. A 20 percent increase in session time per day, per week is the most you should do for the first month or so. So, if you were exercising for 15 minutes per day to start with, you should only bump that up to 18 or 20 minutes per day for the next week. Then the following week you can increase that to 20 or 25 minutes per day, and so on.

There is an exception to this: if you started out with bouts of less than 10 minutes due to a lack of conditioning, then you should increase the duration of your sessions to 10 or 15 minutes per bout as soon as you've improved your fitness enough to do so. The real health benefits of exercise start to kick in at around that 10 to 15 minute threshold,[3] so that's why I'm promoting it as a good short-term goal. It's impossible for me to guess how quickly you might be able to work up to that. There are truly hundreds of physical variables at play, but you and your trainer or physician can figure out what constitutes a safe progression for you.

There is no maximum limit to the amount of time you should spend exercising. According to the National Weight Control Registry, which tracks more than 10,000 individuals who have lost at least 30 pounds and kept the weight off for one year or more, 90 percent of the individuals who made the list exercise for *an hour or more every day*![4] Adding time to your workouts is a great way to burn more calories and accelerate your weight loss. As you add minutes onto your workout, your level of effort generally doesn't decrease. The same is not true of exercise intensity. For most people, as intensity increases, the amount of time spent exercising decreases. So take advantage of those beautiful days and go for long walks or bicycle rides. If you're exercising indoors, then watching a favorite show or listening to a podcast can help you lengthen your workout time. If you're participating in a class or lifting weights at the gym and you get there early or find you have some extra time afterward, jump on a cardio machine for 10 to 15 minutes. Again, don't focus too much on your level of effort here; just focus on getting in those extra minutes and congratulate yourself when you do!

## Intensity: Break a Sweat!

If fitness level is not a limiting factor for you but time is, then you'll probably want to crank up the intensity at this point. Another word to describe intensity is *effort*, and there are a number of factors you can manipulate that will change your effort level.

Pace, or speed, is the variable that usually comes to mind first, and the one that walkers, cyclists, and joggers usually focus on. All other things remaining equal, any increase in pace will place greater demands on the body, requiring you to expend more calories and resulting in greater physiological responses by the body systems (i.e., better health benefits).

Incline is another way to instantly make your workload harder. An increase of as little as 0.5 percent can make a noticeable difference. If you typically exercise outdoors, then changing your route will vary the incline you traverse. If you walk or jog on a treadmill, it will almost certainly have a range of inclines you can choose from. I recommend you not increase the incline by more than 2 percent when starting out, and don't keep it set there for the entire workout. Doing so can place a lot of strain on the ankles and knees. Following a "rolling hill" program (in which the machine periodically adjusts the incline up or down automatically), or manually raising and lowering the incline every couple of minutes is a good way to start adding intensity to your workouts.

On stationary bicycles and elliptical machines, instead of adding an incline, you will likely have a resistance setting. Increasing the resistance imitates the feeling of cycling or striding uphill. The machine is just mechanically simulating this rather than changing the actual cant of the surface you are on. Some elliptical machines have an incline feature as well, which imitates the motions of a stair climber. You don't have to worry about gradually introducing resistance on stationary cycles and ellipticals like you do with incline on a treadmill because there is little risk of injury. It is likely, however, that you will fatigue more quickly with a steady resistance increase, so just know that you probably won't be able to go as long at the higher resistance.

The technique I mentioned of repeatedly raising the incline for a couple of minutes, then lowering it back down is one version of a technique known as interval training. When you first set out to increase the intensity of your workouts, it's a great idea to utilize intervals as a way of burning more calories and getting fitter. Because you're only doing them for relatively short periods of time, you can go pretty hard during the work phases of an interval session. This is great for making major improvements in your aerobic fitness, and can eventually allow you to train at an overall higher intensity for a sustained period of time. An example of an interval workout would be something like this:

Step 1. Warm-up: Work at a light to moderate pace for three to five minutes. By the end of the warm-up, you should be at your usual level of effort.

Step 2. Work Phase: For 30 to 120 seconds, work at a fairly high intensity. The duration of this phase depends on how hard you're working, which depends on your current level of fitness and your goal for the workout. (A trainer can help you figure this out.)

Step 3. Recovery Phase: For 60 to 240 seconds, slow back down (or decrease the incline or resistance) to your previous effort level. By the end of the recovery phase, you should feel ready to go hard again.

Repeat Steps 2 and 3 for the determined number of times. It's a good idea to start with four or five cycles, but you can build it up to eight or ten as you get more fit.

*Step 4. Cool Down: End with a cool-down phase that brings you from a moderate to a very easy level of effort over three to five minutes. Your rate of breathing should slow back down, close to your base rate.*

In addition to interval workouts, when you feel you're ready to take your effort level up a notch, you should periodically do some continuous effort workouts at an intensity that's just slightly above what you've been doing. For example, if you had been spending the past few months walking at 3.0 miles per hour and started off doing 15 minutes of walking, then slowly increased the duration of your walks up to 30 minutes, you should now walk for 30 minutes at a pace of 3.2 or 3.3 miles per hour. This type of workout taxes your body's systems in different ways than the interval workouts, so it's a good idea to do some of both types each week.

I'd like to warn you here about the tendency that new exercisers have of beginning their workout program at the wrong effort level. Up to now, I've urged you to really take it slow, and to only do what you feel comfortable doing. But for many, starting out *too slowly* can be a problem. There is a delicate balance between what is too difficult and what is not difficult enough. For many individuals, the determining factor is time. If you don't have much time to spend exercising (20 minutes per day, let's say), you may want to ramp up your intensity sooner than someone who can dedicate 40 minutes or more. The reason is the calorie balance—working out at an easy pace for 20 minutes doesn't burn many calories at all. So if you're always short on time, then your initial goal should be to build up intensity and exercise continuously for your entire available time period.

An aerobic workout of at least 15 minutes provides nearly the same health benefits as a longer workout of the same intensity, so that's good, but remember that you're also doing this as part of your weight-loss effort. If you have more time to spend exercising, then you should use it! In terms of pure calorie burn, finding the right balance between time and intensity is a tricky thing. You actually get more bang for your calorie-burning buck by increasing the intensity, but there are other things to consider—chief among them is safety, since adding time to your workout is the safest way to get fitter.

Another big issue with higher intensity is the psychological toll it can take. As you start feeling a bit more fit, you'll probably get excited and want to take your workouts to the next level. And then a couple of weeks later, the excitement will have worn off and your workouts will feel harder. You might start to dread them, and then you might start to skip them. So don't get overly hung up on increasing intensity. If picking up the pace or adding hills or resistance makes you start disliking something you previously enjoyed, bring it back down a notch. Remember that the best exercise is the one you will do consistently! We'll revisit the topic of intensity in chapter 10, when you might feel more ready to push yourself a bit harder.

##  Exercise 22: Step Your Workouts Up a Notch.

For this exercise, pick the *one* FIT variable you want to focus on and spend the next couple of weeks *gradually* taking your workouts to the next level. You probably shouldn't try to make all of your workouts longer or more intense. In fact, depending on your personal level of fitness, your love (or hatred) of exercise, your current motivation level, and the time you have available, you might only modify two or three of your workouts each week. It can be good, both mentally and physically, to have "hard" workout days and "easy" workout days, or "long" workout days and "short" workout days. In your journal, decide which variable you'll change and make the appropriate adjustments to your weekly calendar. Also think about what things you might need to have with you that you didn't before. Will you need to carry water now because you're exercising for a longer period of time? Will you need a sweat towel and a shower kit because you'll be working at a higher intensity? Think of any potential barriers to your new exercise behaviors, and plan right now how you'll set yourself up to overcome them.

## Character Example

Because of Bob's health-risk profile, increasing the intensity of his workouts isn't an option yet. He has been doing a pretty good job of getting in 15 minutes of exercise on six or seven days per week, so he decides to try increasing the duration of his workouts by a few minutes each day. Here's what Bob writes in his journal:

*Exercise 22: Increase the Duration of My Workouts.*

*I've been pretty successful at getting in some exercise almost every day, and I'm finally not feeling so spent at the end of 15 minutes. I've mostly been walking outside after work, but twice last week I did some light strength training at the work gym (after everyone else had gone home for the day). I'm going to stick with lower-intensity workouts, but I'll increase the time I spend walking from 15 minutes to 20 minutes, and I'll add one additional strength exercise to my routine this week. Here's what I'll need to do in order to meet this goal:*

- *Walking: I'll walk five days this week for 20 minutes each time. Looking at my calendar for the week, I'm going to have to get in three of these walks before work, so that means waking up earlier. The temperature is dropping and it's not getting light out until I'm halfway to work now, so I'll also have to bundle up a bit more and wear some reflective clothing. I'm going to set my alarm seven minutes earlier on my walking mornings to be sure I have enough time to dress properly and get in my five extra minutes.*
- *Strength Training: I'm actually looking forward to this part of the goal! I've enjoyed my strength-training workouts in the gym at work, and I can't wait to add a shoulder exercise to my routine. I'll do a set of dumbbell presses at the beginning of my routine, before the bicep and tricep exercises.*
- *I feel pretty confident and won't mind working out with others in the gym as long as I bring my good set of workout clothes. I'll add a note about that to my daily reminder app on the days I plan to exercise at work.*

## Character Example

Ellen's fitness level doesn't pose a big health risk, and in fact, she would like to get in better shape for her job, so she decides to focus primarily on the intensity of her exercise sessions for the next two weeks. Here's the plan she creates:

*Exercise 22: Step Up the Intensity of My Workouts.*

*I've been pretty successful at getting in some exercise every day so far—I only missed one day out of the last nine. My workouts have consisted of mostly walking, with some very short spurts of jogging and some basic calisthenics. For the next two weeks, I want to incorporate more jogging into my walks and do more sets of push-ups, squats, and crunches to start getting my strength to where it should be. Here's my plan for each workout:*

- *Walk/Jog: I'll start with 5 minutes of progressively faster walking to warm up, then jog for 30 seconds and walk for 1 minute until I've been going for 20 minutes, and then I'll walk slowly for 5 minutes to cool down.*
- *Calisthenics: I'll increase the number of sets of push-ups, squats, and crunches I do on Tuesdays and Thursdays from two to three sets. I'll also try to add one or two more repetitions to each set as I am able.*

*I'll definitely be working up a sweat, so if I do these workouts at the police station before my shift, I'll have to shower afterward. I'll be sure to get there plenty early and have my shower kit in my locker.*

# Step Twelve:
# EAT LIKE YOU MEAN IT

We're almost at the point where you'll start tracking your calories and aiming for a daily target number that corresponds to your pounds-per-week weight-loss goal. First, though, it's time for you to shore up your diet and begin strictly following your chosen plan. It's important to note that as you complete this next exercise, you're likely to find one or two things that will be really, really hard for you to change. I don't want you to get hung up on those things right now, so change as many things as you are reasonably able to, and we'll worry about those last few stubborn habits a bit later.

Prior to now, you were just focusing on a few specific dietary behaviors, and giving some minor thought and effort to following your chosen diet on the whole. In this key exercise, you'll go "all in" and commit to following your chosen diet religiously for one full week. Before we get to the exercise, though, I want to discuss one behavior that is key to this process.

## Meal Planning

I like to tell my clients often, "Willpower happens at the grocery store." Once you bring something bad into your home, you've lost the battle—sooner or later it *will* be eaten. I can't stress enough how important it is to plan ahead and make conscious decisions when you are shopping. In addition to the time you spend each week exercising and preparing nutritious meals, you also need to set aside a little time to plan your weekly menu and write an exhaustive but well-crafted shopping list.

It's important that you list every last thing you will need rather than tell yourself you'll grab the staples or the "usual items" after you've picked up everything on your list, because that is bound to leave you roaming the aisles of the grocery store, being tempted by all of those great sales on the end-caps. It's also likely to make you forget something you needed, which will result in another trip to the store, which puts you in front of those tempting choices all over again.

When you first start meal planning, it might take a couple of hours to plan out breakfast, lunch, dinner, and snacks for the next four to seven days, but that's exactly what you should do. If you can afford the shopping time later in the week, I suggest you only plan your menu three or four days in advance, two times per week, because it gives you more flexibility, and it means that your produce will be fresher. You will also be less likely to throw away ingredients that you meant to use up but never did. However, if you can only afford the time for one big shopping trip per week, then plan very carefully, and stick to your plan!

Once you've decided what you want to eat and when, the next step is to take stock of what you have on hand. Be very thorough when you do this. How much brown rice is left in that bag—is it enough for all of the meals you intend to use it in? Are those green beans going to make it to Tuesday, when you plan to have them in your veggie stir-fry? Check the dates on perishables, and give them a sniff and a taste if they're within a few days of expiring. Then make your list, but don't just write down ingredients haphazardly. Decide which store(s) you will be shopping at, and visualize the layout of the store. Then organize your list according to your most direct route through the store. Start with produce, hit dry and canned goods in the middle, and end with frozen items and perishables like fish, dairy, and eggs. If you also need household items (cleaning supplies, toothpaste, pet food, etc.) you can grab those on your way to the check-out because they're usually located near the freezer section. Most importantly, stick to the list! Don't ever buy something because it's on sale or it looks good or you think you're running low on it. This will not only save you money, it will potentially save you many calories from eating foods that were not on your menu plan.

Once you get the groceries home, it's time to go back to your menu plan and see which items you are going to use and on which day. Freeze things you won't eat until later in the week, and securely store dry goods and oils in a cool, dark place. Then it's time to clear off the counter and deal with all of that produce! If you want to work more fruits and vegetables into your diet, the best way to do so is to wash, dry, cut, and pack them into conveniently sized and luggable containers right when you get them home from the store. Rinse the berries and let them air-dry before refrigerating. If you put them in the fridge wet, they're more likely to mold, and if you don't rinse them, you're less likely to grab a handful to snack on when you're mining the fridge for a little something sweet after dinner. I like to keep cherry tomatoes, cucumbers, carrots, and bell peppers on hand as raw veggie snacks. I wash and air-dry the cherry tomatoes and leave them right on the counter where I can see them. Often I'll put them into a bowl rather than leave them in the clamshell package so they're easily accessible and look very appealing. I wash and cut up the cucumber, carrots, and bell peppers, and pack them into storage containers in a little cold water, where they stay fresh for up to a week and are easy to grab.

I don't recommend prewashing lettuces and herbs unless you're very diligent about getting them dry before you pack them into the fridge. They can go bad quickly if left with water clinging to their leaves. I do highly recommend the purchase and daily use of a salad spinner, though, which will make your leafy-green prep so much easier you'll wonder how you ever lived without one! Precut and bagged greens can be a real time-saver, but know that the freshness and quality of those greens can never match a locally grown head of lettuce or bunch of kale. Pre-bagged greens are also more prone to contamination, so be sure to rinse thoroughly before using, even if the bag promises that they are "triple washed, ready to use."

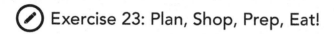 ## Exercise 23: Plan, Shop, Prep, Eat!

The first time you plan and prep your meals, it will probably be pretty time-consuming, but it's crucial to your long-term success, and I promise you'll get much better at it with just a couple weeks of practice. We will break this exercise down into several steps: (1) Start with your dietary reference material close at hand (cookbooks, recipe websites, etc.). (2) Make an extensive meal plan for the next week. Include meals, snacks, and beverages, and pick out specific recipes. (3) Working from your selected recipes, make a list of every ingredient you'll need for your entire meal plan. (4) Take a thorough inventory of which ingredients you have on hand. (5) Write a grocery list based on what you still need to buy. Think about non-food items too, like cleaning supplies, pet supplies, paper products, etc., so that you only need to shop once. (6) Go shopping *and stick to the list*! (7) Right when you get home from the store, prep, package, and put away your ingredients. (8) Spend the next week strictly following your menu plan. (9) Track everything you eat and drink carefully in your food log.

While you should continue tracking calories and grams of fat/protein/carbs, worry less about controlling them at this point—your goal for this exercise is to closely follow your chosen eating plan. If you run into roadblocks that seem too big to tackle (cravings for foods that are not in the plan or extreme dislike of certain foods that are), then give yourself a little wiggle room. This is an exploratory week, designed to get you used to the process of meal planning and smart shopping, and to help you decide whether to stick with the plan you've chosen or try a different one.

## Character Example

Back in Exercise 13, Bob decided to give the higher-protein diet a try. To help guide him, he purchased two cookbooks filled with recipes geared toward a healthy lifestyle, and he bookmarked three websites with recipes from experts (one registered dietitian and two healthy-cooking celebrity chefs). Over the next week, Bob looks for recipes whenever he has a block of 15 minutes here or there. By the time Friday evening rolls around, he's got half his meal plan for the week already done. He finishes it up before he goes to bed Friday night. Here's how Exercise 23 looks for Bob:

*Exercise 23: Plan, Shop, Prep, and Eat!*

*Menu Plan for the Week*

- *Breakfast (M–F): Oatmeal with 1/2 oz. walnuts, 1/2 oz. raisins, cinnamon, and 1/4 cup skim milk; 1 small banana; coffee*
- *Breakfast (Sa–Su): Omelet of 1 egg and 3 egg whites, onions, peppers, and tomatoes; 1 piece whole-grain toast with 1 tsp. butter; coffee*
- *Mid-morning Snack (M–Su): 1/2 oz. almonds; 1 small piece of fresh fruit*
- *Lunch (M–F): Turkey breast, lettuce, tomato, and 1/8 avocado on whole wheat; 1 small apple; water*
- *Lunch (Sa–Su): Vegetarian chili; 1 piece whole-grain bread plain; 1 small orange; water*
- *Afternoon Snack (M–Su): 1 cup raw veggies with 2 tbsp. lite ranch dressing; 3/4 cup Southwest Bean Salad*
- *Dinner (M–F): Large salad with cucumber, tomato, chickpeas, and 2 tbsp. lite dressing; 6 oz. grilled lean chicken or fish; 3/4 cup cooked brown rice or quinoa; water or 12 oz. beer or 6 oz. wine (limit of 4 alcoholic drinks per week)*
- *Dinner (Sa–Su): Large salad with cucumber, tomato, chickpeas, and 2 tbsp. lite dressing; 3/4 cup cooked whole-wheat pasta with ground turkey Bolognese; 2 oz. whole-wheat bread with 1/2 tbsp. butter*

- *Dessert (M –Su): 1 cup fresh pineapple or 3 Medjool dates or 1/2 cup low-calorie frozen yogurt with 1 tbsp. slivered almonds*
- *Nighttime Snack (M –Su): 2 cups popcorn, air-popped, with 1 tbsp. butter and 1/4 tsp. salt*

Bob makes a list of everything he'll need to make the meals on his menu:

| | |
|---|---|
| *Oatmeal* | *1 can Kidney Beans* |
| *Walnuts* | *2 cans Chickpeas* |
| *Raisins* | *Lite Ranch Dressing* |
| *Cinnamon* | *1 Cucumber* |
| *Skim Milk* | *Cherry Tomatoes* |
| *Bananas* | *Baby Carrots* |
| *Coffee* | *Chili Powder* |
| *Eggs* | *Cumin* |
| *2 Onions* | *Cayenne Pepper* |
| *2 Peppers* | *Brown Rice* |
| *3 Tomatoes* | *2 pkgs. Chicken Breasts* |
| *Whole-Grain Bread* | *12 oz. Salmon fillet* |
| *Almonds* | *6 oz. Tilapia fillet* |
| *Apples* | *Whole-Wheat Pasta* |
| *Oranges* | *Ground Turkey* |
| *Pineapple* | *Medjool Dates* |
| *Eggs* | *Frozen Yogurt* |
| *Turkey Breast* | *Dried Oregano* |
| *Lettuce* | *Fresh Basil* |
| *Avocado* | *Popcorn* |
| *2 cans Diced Tomatoes* | *Butter* |

Next Bob takes a thorough inventory of what he has on hand, then makes a grocery list, thinking about the layout of the store he normally shops at:

| | |
|---|---|
| 1 bunch Bananas | 2 cans Chickpeas |
| 2 Onions | 1 can Kidney Beans |
| 2 Bell Peppers | 1 pkg. Whole-Wheat Pasta |
| Bag of Apples | 1 loaf Whole-Grain Bread |
| Bag of Oranges | 1/2 gallon Skim Milk |
| 1 Pineapple | 1 pkg. Butter |
| Bag of Baby Carrots | 1 lb. Ground Turkey |
| Cherry Tomatoes | 2 pkgs. Chicken Breasts |
| 1 Cucumber | 12 oz. Salmon |
| 1 Avocado | 6 oz. Tilapia |
| 3 heads Lettuce | 1 pint Frozen Yogurt |
| 1 bunch Basil | Toilet Paper |
| 1 pkg. Medjool Dates | Dog Treats |
| 1 bag Walnuts | Dishwasher Detergent |
| 2 cans Diced Tomatoes | |

Bob does the shopping on Saturday and is surprised at how hard it is for him to stick to the list. He's tempted several times to buy things he sees on sale, but he makes himself adhere to items on his list. When he gets the groceries home, he puts away the canned and dried goods, then turns his attention to the poultry and fish. He repackages the chicken breasts into single servings so he doesn't have to thaw and refreeze the whole package and does the same with the salmon fillet by cutting it in half. Next he washes and cuts his fresh veggies and cuts the whole pineapple into bite-sized chunks, packaging them into six small snack-sized containers. Bob is ready for the week ahead!

At the end of his week, he reviews his food log and writes the following entry in his notebook:

*This week was a little tough at times, but I think this diet plan is something I can stick with. I ate often enough and large enough portions that I didn't feel hungry, but I struggled with cravings almost every day. I really wanted to eat a hamburger all week, and I finally gave in on Saturday night when we were out for dinner. I skipped the fries, though, and had a salad with lite dressing, so I didn't feel too bad about it—until I put it in my food log later! Turns out, there are lots of calories and fat in a half-pound bar burger. At nighttime, I struggled to only eat 1/2 cup of frozen yogurt, and actually found that the dates were more satisfying because they are so sweet. It was surprising to see how many more calories I took in on the weekend, even though it felt like I was hardly splurging at all. But between the beer and the pasta and the extra serving of bread and butter, it adds up quickly. Still, this is a world better than the way I've been eating. I'm going to stick with this eating plan.*

At this point, it's important to note that your experience might be different from Bob's. If you had trouble sticking with your initial healthy eating plan, then make adjustments or choose a different plan and repeat this exercise until you find one that you can stick with for the long term. Remember that it takes time to develop a taste for new foods and to overcome cravings. Be patient with yourself and don't get frustrated. It's important that you get this crucial exercise right before moving on.

# Step Thirteen:
# COUNT YOUR CALORIES

Once you've found the eating plan that works best for you, it's time to plug real numbers into the formula and determine your daily calorie target in order to achieve your weekly weight-loss goal. It is very important that you read the next few paragraphs before you get busy worrying about the numbers, though, because this is the part of the program where you can crash and burn if you don't proceed with great caution.

First, let's consider why counting calories is necessary. At this point, your eating and exercise habits are already looking a lot better than they were a few weeks ago, so is it really necessary to track calories? The answer is actually different for different people. Some of you would do just fine from here on out if you simply follow your healthy eating plan and continue exercising daily. But some others might not lose a single pound by following that approach. The reason is that some people are just better at inherently knowing how much of which types of foods to eat in order to lose weight. Other people will think they're eating healthier, and they very well may be, but they're still taking in too many calories for their gender, age, height, and body type. At this point, it's better for everyone to be on the safe side and track calories for at least two solid weeks.

What you're looking for in this next exercise is where to pick your battles. Is portion control your big problem, or are infrequent but very-high-calorie "treats" your potential downfall? Are you a carboholic, or can you not resist bacon and sausage? Your biggest dietary obstacles will be revealed to you in this next exercise.

There are two risks you run when completing this exercise, and you need to be aware of them so you can avoid them. The first is the risk of adverse psychological effects that can result from calorie restriction. Remember earlier when I talked about how many people hate being told what to do? Well, telling yourself to only eat X number of calories per day can be a pretty big deal, and many people respond by rebelling, whether they consciously know it or not. For this reason, I suggest that most of you count your calories for two weeks and *two weeks only*. By knowing that there is an end to the imposed calorie restriction, you'll be less likely to rebel and more likely to stick with your diet plan. However, if you find that counting calories is the only way to keep you on track, and if you don't feel that the restriction presents an issue for you, then it's fine (and advised, in fact) to continue beyond the two weeks. Each person must make this decision on his or her own.

The second risk this exercise presents can be even more dangerous: cutting your calories way too much. Using a couple of our characters as examples, let me illustrate a shocking scenario. If Bob wants to lose one pound per week, he'll plug his numbers into his food log and it will tell him that he can eat approximately 2,740 calories per day. However, if Cindy wants to lose one pound per week, she can only eat 1,560 calories per day. If Cindy has been used to eating around 2,900 calories per day, imagine what it's going to be like for her to cut her daily calorie intake nearly in half!

This is why it's so important for Cindy, and for you, to choose a realistic weight-loss goal. I recommend that you not cut your daily calorie intake by more than one-third of your previous daily average. Even if this means super slow weight loss, it's better than a more drastic reduction. The reason why is that you need to create a "positive feedback loop" for yourself throughout this process: the benefits you realize *must* outweigh the sacrifices you make. If cutting your calories by a little means you only lose a little weight, but you aren't hungry, tired, crabby, etc., then you will be enjoying success with relatively little pain. You're more likely to stick with the program in that case. If you cut your calories drastically, though, then the first week you fail to hit your calculated weight-loss goal, the chances of you giving up are very high. Remember that this is a long-term effort, and the way to win is to stay in the game—consistency is key!

# ✎ Exercise 24: Determine Your Daily Calorie Target, Then Stick to It.

Now you'll plug your numbers into your food log program or an online calorie calculator. You'll enter your current weight, goal weight, and target rate of weight loss in pounds per week. If you're doing a pen-and-paper food log, you can use the calculators to determine your daily calorie target at http://www.calculator.net/calorie-calculator.html or http://www.healthyweightforum.org/eng/calculators/calories-required/.

Be sure to get an accurate current weight—your weight might have changed since the last time you checked it, and it's the most important piece of your calorie formula.

## Character Example

As discussed above, Cindy would need to cut her calories drastically in order to lose one pound per week, so she decides that half pound per week is just fine. Here's how her food log settings page looks after she enters her specific details:

| Personal Information | | | |
|---|---|---|---|
| Current Weight: | 192 lbs. | | |
| Goal Weight: | 150 lbs. | | |
| Height: | 5 ft. | 8 in. | |
| Gender: | male | X female | |
| Date of Birth: | September | 1 | 1985 |
| Normal Daily Activity Level (check one) | | | |
| X Sedentary | Spend most of the day sitting (e.g. bank taller, desk job) | | |
| | Spend a good part of the day on your feet (e.g. teacher, salesman) | | |
| | Spend a good part of the day doing some physical activity (e.g. waitress, mailman) | | |
| | Spend most of the day doing heavy physical activity (e.g. bike messenger, carpenter) | | |
| Exercise | | | |
| Weekly Goal | 0 workouts/week | 0 minutes/workout | |
| Preferred Tracking | | | |

| Goal | | |
|---|---|---|
| What is your goal? | Lose .5 pounds per week | |
| **Nutritional Goals** | **Target** | |
| Net Calories | 1,810 calories/day | |
| Carbs/Day | 226.0 g | |
| Fat/Day | 60.0g | |
| Protein/Day | 91.0g | |

Note that Cindy is still not taking credit for any exercise. Rather, she'll try to hit her calorie target each day through diet alone, and any extra calories she burns through exercise will move her toward her goal that much faster.

Of course, figuring out how many calories you can eat each day is the easy part; limiting yourself to that many calories is the hard part. Keep in mind the example from earlier in the book about the individual who "saved" her calories up throughout the day so that she could indulge later on. Don't be that person. Rather, aim to spread your allotted calories out over the course of the day so that your energy levels stay steady and you don't find yourself starving and ready to eat whatever you can get your hands on. Rely on vegetables and a little fruit to fill the hours between your meals. They'll fill you up without adding many calories. Drink lots of water throughout the day too. Often perceived hunger is actually thirst, so not only will water fill your stomach for a while, but it may turn off the hunger signal from your brain entirely.

You'll likely have a time of day or a situation that is more difficult for you. It's important during those times that you immediately focus on your goals, and then employ the tactics you devised in Exercises 20 and 21 for overcoming those particular barriers. Know this, though: if you are losing weight, you *will* be hungry. However, the amount by which you initially cut calories will determine whether your hunger will be too big an obstacle for you. If you're losing weight at a reasonable rate, the hunger will be manageable and you won't often give in to cravings or other temptations. However, if you're creating a calorie deficit that is too large, this will be a constant and unpleasant battle for you. Even if you are losing weight at a slightly faster pace, you'll be much more susceptible to slipping into a lapse at the first sign of trouble. Remember the positive feedback loop—slow down and be patient. Remind yourself that you're not on a short-term diet this time; you're doing this for the rest of your life. You need to create a program for yourself that is sustainable. Sure, once you've lost the weight it will be a lot less work to keep it off, but you will still maintain a healthy lifestyle—you are changing who you are and how you live. You are becoming the thin, fit, healthy person you have always wanted to be.

## Chapter Eight

# THE FINAL PIECES OF THE PUZZLE

You've learned a lot so far. You've changed the way you think about yourself, the way you talk to yourself, the way you picture yourself. You've made an iron-clad commitment to losing weight—not just "this time," but for a lifetime. You've acknowledged that you will be a different person once you've successfully made this lifestyle change, and you've committed to this for the long term, not just for some temporary period of time. You've started to radically change not only what you eat but also how you think about food. You're exercising almost every day. You've learned strategies for overcoming the many barriers you'll face, but there's one more key piece of information you need in order to join the ranks of the successful 20 percent: you need to learn how to fail.

## No One Is Perfect

There are many things you can't predict about your weight-loss journey, but one thing is certain: you will encounter setbacks along the way. You'll have a bad day here and there that will move you backward instead of forward; you'll have a string of bad days that will cause a short lapse; you might become ill or injured and have to deal with a more long-term setback. Sometimes the reasons for your setbacks will be beyond your control, and other times you'll simply make poor decisions. The important thing is to expect these setbacks and to view them as temporary when they do happen.

Injuries and illness can be extremely difficult to deal with—they are things that happen to you and usually are not the product of your own actions, and they often last for days or even weeks. This can easily lead to frustration, and frustration can sap motivation, especially if the episode is prolonged. I have found that the key to dealing with illness and injury is to take a short period (one or two days) of true rest, and then to ask myself, "What am I still able to do?" There is almost always *something* you can do.

In my mid-thirties, I had the brilliant idea of having bunion surgery on both of my feet at the same time. As a result, I was left scooting from the bed to the bathroom on my butt for two weeks, and then spent the next month hobbling awkwardly in double walking casts. But I still exercised! I devised a workout I could do in bed. It was heavy on crunches, knee push-ups, and leg lifts (and those bandages and casts were kind of heavy!), but it was enough to fill 15 or 20 minutes and I did it nearly every day. At the end of my six-week recovery, I was happy to find that I hadn't lost much muscle tone, and I hadn't gained any weight (obviously I had to adjust my diet a bit).

If your injury is severe and you can't exercise at all, then you can use your usual workout time to take your meal planning and healthy cooking skills to the next level. If you're totally bed-ridden, you can ask your caregivers to feed you nutritious salads and soups and whole grains, and you can read up on the latest exercise and nutrition information.

Lapses are more common than illness or injury, and are often tied to times of increased stress, changes in your routine, and so forth. When the kids first start their summer vacation; during the holidays; in the weeks leading up to a big work deadline—these are all times when your healthy routine can be thrown off. You miss a workout; you grab a less-than-healthy meal on the road. One day turns into two, and pretty soon it's been two weeks and your weight loss comes grinding to a halt. This is a lapse, but it is *not* a relapse into your old habits, *unless you allow it to become one.*

Guess what your most important weapon against relapse is? It's your brain! You need to return to Step 2 and *believe* that you will lose weight. A 2012 study published in the *Journal of Experimental Psychology* found that when individuals were facing a weight-loss plateau or lapse period, those who received coaching to help them believe their body weight was something they could change regained much less weight than those who were given only information on diet and exercise.[1] By not getting caught up in "all or nothing" thinking, and by truly believing in your power to change your body, you'll get back on track sooner.

Of course, it is also important to do some investigative work about what caused the setback in the first place and then make a plan for how to avoid the same kind of setback in the future. To do this, you have to acknowledge lapses when they occur and be honest with yourself by taking ownership and not blaming external circumstances. Instead, acknowledge that you failed to adapt to those circumstances, and then formulate a plan for how you'll do better the next time. Go back to Exercises 19 through 21 and identify the particular obstacles that have crept up during your setback, classify them by type, and practice strategies for defeating them.

Possibly the worst kind of setback is one that involves your own poor decisions. This is because those decisions are often accompanied by guilt, denial, or shame, and those emotions are not useful to your progress. It's easy to make poor decisions—you get caught up in the moment and tell yourself, "Hey, I've been good for so long, I deserve this!" But truthfully, you are choosing to take an action that is moving you further away from your goal. Everyone will make those kinds of choices at one time or another, but it's important to be honest in each instance and identify that it *is* a choice. Excuses come in many forms and are as useless to you as guilt and shame. In fact,

**Your success in this effort will be inversely proportionate to the number of excuses you make.**

So, even though you will not always make *good* decisions, you should strive to at least make *conscious* decisions. If you're skipping a workout or eating something unhealthy or falling into a day of self-pity and negative self-talk, then just own up to it. Consciously say, "This is what I'm doing." And say it right then, in that moment. Don't wait until after the party when you're lying in bed unable to sleep from the guilt. Take responsibility for your decision right when you make it, ensuring that one bad decision won't cascade into a string of them. Taking responsibility is a necessary action you will need to master in this process. The reason why you make a poor dietary decision is often less important than simply acknowledging that you are consciously choosing to do so. This gives you responsibility and ownership; it makes you the person in control rather than a victim of circumstance. If you repeatedly choose to ignore your behaviors until after the fact, you will never be able to change them.

## Step Fourteen:
# PLAN FOR MINOR SETBACKS AND FAILURES

This step is all about getting you back on track, no matter what has caused you to slip in the first place. The process of logically examining your failures so that you don't repeat them in the future is one of the most important skills you can learn. No one is perfect at anything, ever. What distinguishes the successful people in any arena is their ability to adapt and improve.

## ✏ Exercise 25: Write a Script That Will Get You Back on Track.

This exercise presumes an important fact: that you *know setbacks will occur*. This exercise is not only about damage control (what you do after the fact), but it is also about preemptive planning. Don't wait until you've slipped up to come to this exercise. Rather, write up a bare-bones outline for yourself now, so that when you do have a moment of failure, you'll know exactly what to do. This exercise gives you a plan for how you'll deal with your lapses before they even happen.

While it's impossible to predict specifically when, where, or how you will falter, the path to getting back on track is virtually the same in any circumstance. First, you'll need to do a deep analysis of what happened—examine what the circumstances were, down to the smallest detail; what your emotions were like; whether you were under pressure from outside forces, under great stress, or lacking motivation. Then you'll need to ask yourself what you can change *right now* to keep this minor setback from becoming a more long-term relapse into previous poor habits. It's important not to delay this exercise more than a day or two. Once you've had your moment of guilt or self-pity, or (more desirable) an hour or two of nonjudgmental contemplation, pick up your notebook and write out a script that does these three things:

1. Acknowledge what happened.
2. Take responsibility for what happened.
3. Lay out a clear path forward both for getting back to your new, positive behaviors and for preventing a similar setback in the future.

## Character Example

Ellen writes out a quick outline that she'll use whenever she gets stuck.

*Exercise 25: Write a Script That Will Get You Back on Track.*
1. *State what happened.*
2. *Figure out why it happened.*
   a. *What were my emotions like? My stress level?*

   b. *Was anyone else involved, and in what way?*

   c. *Was my motivation low? If so, why?*

3. *Brainstorm ways to get out of this slump.*

   a. *Set a time-bound deadline.*

   b. *List specific actions to take.*

4. *Plan how I can prevent this from happening again in the future.*


*A few days after drawing up her outline, Ellen has a bad day, and not only blows her calorie target by a few hundred calories but skips her workout too. She goes back to Exercise 25 and fills in the details:*


1. *State what happened.*

   *This was an awful day! I overslept and rushed off to work with no breakfast and without packing a lunch. It was a busy day at work, and I didn't have time to eat until almost one o'clock, when I hit a fast-food drive-through. I figured that since I didn't eat breakfast, I could have whatever I wanted for lunch, so I got a combo meal with a soda. By the time I got home, I felt too tired and upset to bother with exercise or cooking, so I ordered a pizza and sat on the couch and ate two-thirds of it while I watched TV. This has been a total waste of a day.*

2. *Figure out why it happened.*

   a. *Emotions and stress level: I was in a bad mood all day, stressed out because I had overslept. I used this as an excuse to justify my poor choices.*

   b. *Was anyone else involved, and in what way? Nope, this one was all me!*

   c. *Was my motivation low? If so, why? I have been feeling a little whiny the past few days. I overslept this morning because I was up in the middle of the night for over an hour. I'm worried about the department's physical readiness test coming up next month. Boy, is this ever a bad way to deal with that!*

3. *Brainstorm ways to get out of this slump.*

   a. *Set a time-bound deadline. I'm starting fresh tomorrow morning.*

   b. *List specific actions to take. I'll go to bed right after this and double check that my alarm is on the loudest setting. Tomorrow morning I'll have my usual breakfast and pack a healthy lunch. I'll bring extra snacks in case I end up having to work past the end of my shift. I'll work out at the gym before I come home, no matter what. I already have my exercise clothes there, ready to go.*

4. *Plan how I can prevent this from happening again in the future.*

> *I should have sensed something like this was coming. I haven't been focused on my goals as much as I should be lately, and my motivation has been low. It's not surprising that I used this little mishap as an excuse to totally ditch my healthy habits. In the future, I need to check in with my emotions more often and work to keep my attitude positive and my motivation high. I should read my list of motivators and my positive word picture at least twice a week, so they are fresh in my mind. I should also buy some healthy ready-to-go meals and snacks so that even when I'm running late I have something to grab on my way out the door. I know they aren't as good as my home-cooked food, but they're a lot better than the drive-through combo meal!*

This is an exercise you'll probably do many, many times. Your goal, however, should be to only do it once for each specific lapse and not live through the same setbacks time and again. If you're honest with yourself and understand the true reason why the setback happened, you can work to implement effective strategies for prevention (and shouldn't find yourself making the same mistakes over and over again). If you do keep making the same mistakes, then I recommend that you find a coach or a therapist to help you work through your toughest, most deep-seated issues.

## Some Things to Watch Out For

Some people have certain tendencies that make lapses more likely to occur, or more damaging or longer lasting when they do happen. These tendencies are called cognitive distortions, and they represent patterns of thought that are out of sync with the reality of a situation. Keep an eye out for these thought patterns, and take quick action against them when you recognize them.

### All-or-Nothing Thinking

People who participate in all-or-nothing thinking see things in black and white. They are either a success or a failure. They've either stuck to the diet or they haven't. The truth is that each situation usually contains a mix of both components and the exact proportion of the mixture changes from situation to situation and from day to day. You succeed at times and fail at others, and you succeed at some *things* and fail at others. You do a good job of sticking to your diet one day, but not quite as well the next, or you succeed in staying on track from morning until evening, but then divert a little late at night. When these small moments of failure occur, it's irrational to categorize yourself as "failing" or as "a failure."

Thinking of diet and exercise in terms of "rules" that you have either followed or broken is another way you can fall into all-or-nothing thinking. The more consistently you stick to your program, the more quickly you will reach your weight-loss goals, but straying here and there does not mean you'll never reach them. By believing that you *will* succeed despite setbacks, you put the momentum back on your side.

### Overgeneralization

When someone overgeneralizes, they see a failure in one small area as an indicator that they have failed or will fail entirely. They assume that a negative pattern exists when only a single negative event has occurred. A thought like, "I'll never be able to turn down dessert (fried foods, pizza, etc.)," after one instance of giving in to temptation is an example of this cognitive distortion. If you catch yourself saying something similar to that, back up and examine the facts: you didn't resist that temptation this time, but that has no bearing on what you will do the next time. Take a moment to hit the reset button and plan how you will do better next time.

### Mental Filters (Biased Thinking)

A filter is something that allows certain things to pass through while discarding others. A biased mental filter allows negative thoughts to rattle around inside your head while the positive thoughts are downplayed or disregarded altogether. When you allow a biased mental filter to shift your focus more on your failures than on your successes, negative thinking is the result. You spent a lot of time early on in Exercises 3 and 4 getting rid of this negative thinking. Don't let a biased mental filter distort the facts: You are becoming the fit, thin person you want to be, regardless of how many small failures or setbacks you encounter along the way. Your successes far outnumber your failures, and they deserve to be given equal or greater attention from you.

The important thing to remember about this step is that you will have setbacks, so you should expect them and have a plan in place to deal with them. While setbacks do slow your progress toward your goal, nothing can *stop* that progress except for your decision to quit. Learning from your mistakes so that you don't repeat them is the surest way for you to continue moving toward your weight-loss goal. Have patience and compassion for yourself and don't judge, but be firm too—don't allow yourself to slip back into the same lapses time after time.

# Step Fifteen:
# NOW DO IT ALL OVER AGAIN. AND AGAIN.

By now you should have an idea of what this process looks like over the long term. You will make positive behavior changes, and you'll sustain those changes long enough so that they become habits. You'll experience lapses and have to back up and reestablish those habits. In the meantime, you'll target new behaviors and work toward making those changes feel like second nature.

Before I get any further, I'd like to talk a bit about how long it's likely to take for those habits to really set in. The truth is, there is no way to predict how long it will take, but it's probably a lot longer than you were hoping. In an article published in a 2010 issue of the *European Journal of Social Psychology*, researchers found that the amount of time to form a habit varied widely from person to person, ranging from 18 to more than 200 days, with the average being 66 days.[2] Habit formation can depend on many variables, including your personality type, the number of distractors in your life (stress, conflict, a busy schedule, etc.), the difficulty level of the target behavior, and the level of importance you give it. So if you've been moving pretty quickly through the exercises in this book, then you might be finding it tough to stick to all of your new habits right about now. That's okay. When a setback occurs, just remember to acknowledge it, evaluate it, and plan for how to do better moving forward.

From this point on, the order in which you do things (like making further changes to your diet or exercise habits, working on stress management, or getting more sleep, etc.) is up to you. Now is the time to really evaluate how solidly you've incorporated the first few key habits of your new lifestyle, and to go back and do a little more work on the ones that aren't quite up to par. This is where the real work gets done. Glossing over something and assuming that it'll "just come eventually" will not do you any favors.

If you've been struggling with sticking to your eating plan and hitting your daily calorie target (Exercise 24), then you'll need to revisit not only that exercise but possibly also Exercises 13 and 23, where you chose your dietary plan and then committed to it. If you find that you're missing a lot of workouts, then you'll need to go back to Exercise 16 and use the problem-solving strategies you've learned to figure out how you're going to start exercising every day. From here on, you need to check in with yourself *every day* and be honest about how you're doing. At this point, you should be able to identify which behaviors are holding you back. You can also determine what barriers are keeping you from changing those behaviors, and you can work through the steps in order to eliminate those things that are standing in your way. Of course it won't be easy! You might need to hire a trainer or a coach or see a therapist or ask your entire support network for help. You might get stuck on one big bad habit for weeks or months. But you'll keep going, because that's how this process works.

In the chapters that follow, I'll give you some practical tips and advice on a range of topics you no doubt have questions about. I'll provide advanced strategies you can use to clean up your diet, and I'll give you a lot of specific information about how you might choose to progress with your exercise program. I'll talk about the roles that sleep and stress can play in weight loss, and I'll give you a few other behavioral tips and strategies you might find useful. But first, take a word of advice: don't rush to change new behaviors until you are comfortable with the changes you've already been working on. If you do, you'll run the risk of letting those hard-fought habits slip away. This failure can lead to some of the cognitive distortions discussed above, and will damage your motivation and halt your momentum. Remember that this is a lifelong process, so you're in no hurry. We each have a set capacity for willpower. Exceed that capacity too many times, and you're likely to give up the whole effort rather than just scale back to something more manageable. Achieving your ultimate weight-loss goal in five years is infinitely better than giving up in frustration and never achieving it at all.

If you need a little motivational reminder, think about this: As you successfully change your habits one by one, you will be doing much more than simply burning more calories than you take in; you'll be rewriting your biological history and rebooting your body! Your brain will send new signals down new pathways, and your body will learn to respond to food and activity in different ways. The sum of your lifestyle behaviors, day after day, will transform your body in ways that no drug has yet been able to do. You will be a living, breathing epigenetic success story!

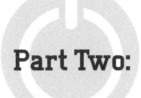

# Part Two:

# TIPS, TRICKS, AND PRACTICAL GUIDANCE

*The essence of permanent behavior change boils down to this:
the will to act, not motivated by a short-term means to an end, but rather
by a permanent, positive attitude that springs from truly believing in your
capabilities, and gratitude for the fact that you possess those capabilities.*

The next few chapters are designed to give you information and tips to help you achieve your ultimate goal. When you're up against a particularly tough barrier, when life throws a mountain of garbage at you, or when you're feeling stuck and don't know what to do, come back to these pages and see if anything you read rings true for you. The ideas, information, and strategies I've included go beyond what you're likely to find in the media or on most online forums and chat groups. You can think of them as advanced strategies—the things you implement after you've already got the basics down or when the basics just aren't cutting it anymore.

## Chapter Nine

# BREAKING THROUGH PLATEAUS

Before I get into some specifics on diet and exercise, I want to talk a bit about the dreaded weight-loss plateau. A plateau is a period of time when nothing happens. You do everything the same as you've been doing for weeks or months, but one day you just stop losing weight. First off, you should know that I have never worked with a client who didn't experience a plateau, regardless of their goals. Athletes trying to get bigger or run faster are every bit as susceptible as regular folks who are just trying to lose weight. There are a few contributing factors at play here, and if you understand and watch out for those factors, you should be able to modify your program and move past your plateaus fairly quickly.

The first factor goes back to what we talked about in the prologue: our bodies are excellent at adapting to new conditions. Adaptation, tolerance, efficiency, call it what you will; the fact is that your body gets used to meeting a certain level of energy demand on a certain number of daily calories in the same way that it gets used to you drinking one beer or three cups of coffee each day. After a while, you don't feel the effects of the beer or the coffee the way you used to. It's the same with exercise—the energy cost of those activities decreases as your body adapts to them, so you burn fewer calories.

The next factor is cruel by design. As you lose weight, your metabolism drops slightly.[1] If you've kept or added some lean muscle mass while you've been losing fat, that drop will happen more slowly. But the truth is that your body weight is the biggest factor in the formula that determines how many calories you burn each day. Where before you were burning 300 calories walking for 20 minutes at a certain pace, now you might only burn 270 calories. Even more worrisome, though, is what your body is doing the other 23.67 hours of the day: it's burning fewer calories because there is less of you to "maintain."

By themselves, these two factors amount to only a few dozen calories per day, but in combination, they can add up to something more significant.

The third factor is the real kick in the pants. Research has shown that failure to adhere to weight-loss strategies, *not* changes in metabolism, is the primary reason for hitting a plateau.[2] In other words, you think you're following your program just as well as you were in the beginning, but in truth you've slipped a little.

Fortunately, there are a couple of strategies that I've found to be very effective against all factors involved with the weight-loss plateau. The first one is that you need to take short breaks from your weight-loss effort. I know this might sound counterintuitive, but once I explain the logic behind it, hopefully it will make more sense.

Don't get too excited. These "breaks" don't give you permission to put your new healthy habits on hiatus and eat whatever you want while channel surfing for hours every evening. Instead, you should continue your habits exactly as you have been, and only slightly adjust your daily calorie balance so that you are maintaining weight rather than losing it. Here's a quick example:

If you had been losing half a pound per week, then you were creating a deficit of 250 calories per day. Let's say that you had been eating 1,800 calories per day in order to create that deficit. Now, for two or three weeks, you should erase that deficit, and strive to simply maintain your current weight. Mathematically, you do this by eating 2,050 calories per day. If you haven't been tracking calories since you finished Exercise 24, then now would be a good time to pick that back up for a week or two. Make sure that you're logging your food and drink diligently, and also *make sure your extra calories are healthy ones*! Add these calories with an extra serving of lean protein or with a little fruit or a lot of vegetables (or some combination of the three). Don't drink your extra calories, and don't splurge on desserts or fatty meats, fried foods, etc. For one thing, you don't want to undo a habit that was probably hard for you to form. More importantly, the way the body processes empty calories is very different from how it processes nutrient-dense foods. Simple sugars and saturated fats are easily converted to fat in the body.[3] Fiber-rich fruits and vegetables and lean sources of protein, on the other hand, are digested more slowly, so your body can use them to sustain your activity rather than converting them to fat.

The timing of these extra calories is also important. Eating them earlier in the day can help ensure that they get used for immediate energy rather than stored as fat. Perhaps the best way to add them is in the form of a post-workout snack. Eating some protein and carbohydrate within 30 minutes of a workout replenishes blood sugar stores and can help your body recover more quickly, which can lead to better fitness gains.[4]

For those who have a lot of weight to lose, I recommend that for every 5 percent of body weight you lose, you take a two-week maintenance break. For those with less to lose, you should take a one- to two-week break for every 5 to 10 pounds lost. Taking these short breaks gets your body used to using more calories again, so that when the break is over and you return to your weight-loss calorie deficit, you should resume losing weight. Another benefit of these breaks is that they give you an opportunity to practice maintaining weight periodically, so that once you reach your final goal weight, you'll already know how to transition into the maintenance phase and be at lower risk for regaining weight.

Another way you can overcome a weight-loss plateau is by changing the demands you place on your body. Here is where exercise becomes an even bigger key to the weight-loss process.

If you've been going along with your regular workouts for several weeks or months and suddenly hit a plateau, that's a good sign that it's time to change up your exercise routine. In most cases, when I say "change," I really mean "intensify," but sometimes merely switching up the kinds of activities you do can get you unstuck. Probably, though, you'll either need to add minutes to your workouts or up your effort level in order to keep your metabolism running high. Now would be a good time to add in some strength-training sessions or cardio intervals if you haven't done so yet. I'll discuss different types of exercise in greater detail and give you some sample workout progressions in the next section, but first I want to be sure you've noticed the one thing I *didn't* recommend for moving past a plateau: cutting more calories from your diet. For many of you, this is a bad idea.

A weight-loss plateau is, in part, the symptom of a stuck metabolism. Your metabolism is stuck because your body has learned how to do more with less. The goal of weight loss is, of course, to teach your body to work with fewer calories than it was before. But at a certain point, reducing calories further becomes harmful to your effort. Each individual is different, so you'll have to assess your own current situation. If you've lost a large amount of weight but you still have a long way to go, then it might make sense to make further reductions to your calorie intake. However, as you work through the last half of your weightloss effort, cutting calories further becomes less and less effective. In fact, as you approach the last five to 10 percent of weight to lose, cutting calories further is likely to disrupt your metabolism, setting you up for future weight regain. If you're approaching your weight-loss goal then I know this can be a scary time, but you have to trust me when I tell you that you're better off keeping your calories the same or even increasing them a little, as discussed above. Of course, this all assumes that you have truly been hitting your target calorie goals regularly—more on that in just a bit.

You should be aware that if you increase calories to the maintenance level, you may gain a pound or two in the first week, but that is an important part of the process of training your body to use all of the calories you're giving it. Don't let fear cause you to cut calories drastically; rather, stick with the maintenance plan for one more week or *very slightly* adjust calories downward.

Defeating the weight-loss plateau requires a delicate balancing act, and you'll have to proceed by using a bit of trial and error. You can try keeping your calorie intake the same while increasing exercise intensity, duration, or frequency; or you can try increasing calories slightly while either keeping exercise the same or increasing intensity, duration, or frequency. Whatever you choose, stick with it for at least a week (two is better) and see if that helps you break through your plateau. Note that if you keep calorie intake the same and increase exercise, this could become your new exercise "standard," so if it's not something you feel is sustainable, then you'll have to explore other options.

Above all, be patient when working through a plateau. No doubt you'll be frustrated, and your frustration is understandable, but it's not a reason to stray from your program. Getting desperate and trying a fad diet, cutting your calories drastically, or forcing yourself to work out like mad will only cause you to burn out and possibly to give up altogether. Work through this barrier wisely, the way you have worked through others. View it as a puzzle that needs solving. Try to remove emotion from the process, and think of it as a scientific experiment. Carefully manipulate the different variables under your control until you find the right combination that puts you back on the path to weight loss.

As you get closer to your final weight-loss goal, your plateaus will become more frequent and they may last longer. That's because your body knows you are approaching your ideal weight, so it's fighting to stay there. Your goal during these late-stage plateaus (which can last for months) should be to maintain all (or nearly all) of the weight you have lost. Give nothing back! Maintain all of the healthy habits you've spent time and effort creating. Consider yourself successful if you are able to do that, and when you're experiencing a period of high motivation, make a renewed effort to lose those final pounds. You'll find some tips for how you can do that in chapters 12 and 13. Before I end this chapter, though, I want you to do one important thing.

## The Reality Check

Remember that third factor, the real reason why people experience weight-loss plateaus? It's because they've let their healthy habits slide a bit.

Losing weight is a long, hard process. Everyone cycles through periods of high and low motivation. Seasons change, holidays come and go, the stressors in your life increase or decrease, and your success follows these ups and downs. A plateau may simply be a down period for you. The only way to know is by taking a close look at how you're doing. If you stopped counting calories after you got comfortable with your new way of eating, now would be a good time to pick it back up for a week or two. It's good to check in with yourself every couple of months and see if you really *are* eating according to plan, or if your little cheats and splurges are adding up to a lot more than you'd thought.

Are you eating late at night again? Stress eating? Are you drinking more than you're acknowledging? Keeping a food log will make it easy for you to see where some of your old habits might be starting to creep back in.

The same goes for exercise. If you haven't upped your intensity, frequency, or duration, or changed up your workout regimen recently, and especially if you've been missing workouts, then it's time to get back on track. Demand more of yourself for a few weeks and see if that doesn't get you moving in the right direction again.

## Chapter Ten

# ALL ABOUT EXERCISE

Up to now, I've mostly just been harping on you to exercise every day. I more or less told you that it doesn't matter what you do, as long as you get and stay in the habit of working out. In chapter 7, you stepped up your weekly workout routine by adjusting frequency, duration, or intensity, but you still might be doing the same one or two things day after day, and you might be wondering if what you're doing is effective. This chapter won't tell you everything you want to know about exercise—thousands of books, articles, and studies have been written on the topic, and there is more being learned every day—but it will be a very good starting point for you. I encourage you to learn more on your own, or better yet, hire a trainer or health coach to give you some professional guidance.

Depending on where you are in your weight-loss journey, you may be using exercise as simply a way to get fitter, or it might be starting to matter in terms of your daily calorie deficits. While I still encourage you to leave exercise out of your calorie counting formula (if you're tracking calories), you'll notice as time goes on that exercise can potentially have a bigger impact on your weight-loss progress than it did at first. By following the tips here, exercise can become a more powerful weapon in your weight-loss arsenal.

### Tell Me What to Do!

As I mentioned back in chapter 5, the best kind of exercise is whatever you'll stick with over time. In this section I'm going to tell you what the most well-rounded type of exercise program looks like, but bear in mind that the most important thing is still that you do *some* activity every day. If you read this whole chapter and still say, "What I'm doing now is the most I am willing or able to do," then I say, keep on keepin' on! Don't let this list of things you "should" do throw you so far out of whack that you end up back at square one, doing nothing. This is a best-case scenario, and if you can approximate some version of it, you will do very well.

## Cardio Is King

In terms of burning calories during exercise, nothing works as well as cardiovascular exercise. In terms of improving your overall fitness and reducing your risk of disease, cardio also ranks number one. So a good exercise program should focus heavily on aerobic activity, giving it priority among your precious weekly exercise minutes. Meta analyses of successful long-term weight-loss participants have shown that over 250 minutes of moderate-intensity cardiovascular exercise per week is associated with significant weight-loss success.[1] That breaks down to around 35 to 45 minutes a day, six or seven days per week. While 250 minutes of cardio per week might sound like an outrageous goal if you've only been exercising for 10 to 20 minutes per day up to now, I encourage you to start adding a few minutes to each workout as you are able. Also, remember that it's fine to break those minutes into more manageable chunks of time throughout the day. As long as the intensity is moderately high and you accumulate 35 to 45 minutes each day, that's all you need!

There are dozens of different kinds of aerobic activities you can do. If you've joined a gym, then you'll have a bevy of machines and probably classes to choose from. I encourage you to try as many different activities as you can, and then rate each one according to which are your favorites and which you really don't like. Then don't bother doing the ones you really don't like for at least a few months. You can try them again later, when you're fitter and more confident, or you don't have to at all—it's up to you.

If you don't have a gym membership, then your options are a little more limited, but there's still a lot you can do. You can walk or jog with minimal money invested; if you own a bicycle, you can ride that; or you could buy a solid but inexpensive piece of cardio equipment, such as a treadmill, stationary cycle, elliptical machine, rowing machine, or stair stepper, for your home. Speaking of stairs, you probably know where to find a few flights, and simply walking up and down them at a slow pace is an extremely good cardiovascular workout.

If you're making your exercise program social, and I recommend that you do, then you can seek out friends, family members, or meet-up groups who participate in (or are willing to take up) activities you are interested in. You can play rec league basketball, volleyball, racquetball, or tennis; you can play Ultimate Frisbee or Frisbee golf; you can join a local walking or running club, or find a group that does trail hiking in your area.

## But Which Exercise Burns the Most Calories?

Maybe you're the sort who will never enjoy exercise, so you figure that if you *have to* do it, you might as well get the most bang for your buck. What can you do to maximize calorie-burning and cardiovascular benefits? Well, you could take up competitive boxing, which burns the most calories per minute (along with other combative forms of mixed martial arts); you could cross-country ski at Olympic racing speeds; you could bicycle at 20 mph or faster; or you could take up jogging.

Running, it turns out, is very energy demanding, even at pretty slow speeds. That's a big part of the reason why it continues to be such a popular activity. In 2011, a survey conducted by the Sporting Goods Manufacturers Association reported that more than 19 million Americans ran 100 days or more that year.[2] In addition to burning a lot of calories, running is also a very social sport, and one that can fuel your competitive drive (even if you'll never reach the middle of the pack, much less win a race). Most runners only ever race against themselves, aiming for a personal record (PR) every time they lace up. The sport can become addictive, but you need to learn the proper running form and a healthy frequency and duration for your runs, or you risk injury. I highly recommend that you work with a personal trainer or running coach, or join a running group for beginners when you get started. It'll help you stay safe and maximize your enjoyment of the sport.

Let's say that boxing, running, and competitive racing in any sport are not your thing. What are some of the next best options? Bicycling can burn quite a few calories—around 60 percent as many as running, but you'll probably burn more on a stationary cycle than you will out on the road because we tend to coast whenever we can on the road. Stairs, stair machines, and elliptical machines will give you a decent calorie burn too, as soon as you're fit enough to ramp up the speed and/or resistance a bit.

Swimming or water aerobics are great options for those who need zero-impact activities due to musculoskeletal issues like past injuries, advanced arthritis, or severe osteoporosis. Some individuals with fibromyalgia and peripheral artery disease have also found that aquatic activities cause less pain than those involving impact forces. You should note, however, that while aquatic exercise (including swimming) is great for the cardiovascular system, it burns fewer calories than exercise at comparable effort levels on dry land. The reason is that much of your bodyweight is supported by the water, so you use less energy to move in the water than you do on land. Also, there is some evidence showing that people get hungrier after swimming than after other forms of exercise.[3] Still, if impact exercises are problematic for you, or if you just want to add variety to your routine, swimming is an excellent option.

There are several good activity calorie calculators online (just type that phrase into your favorite search engine) that will not only give you decent calorie estimates per minute of exercise based on your weight but will give you a big list of activities to try that you might not have considered.

## Going Beyond Cardio

Even though cardiovascular exercise is the most beneficial for burning calories and reducing health risks, you should include a few other important types of exercise in order to have a well-rounded program.

Strength training is important for overall fitness, especially as we get older, because once we reach age thirty or so, our bodies begin to naturally lose muscle mass unless we do something to counter that. By the time you reach forty, if you haven't been strength training, you've most likely lost 7 to 10 percent of your lean muscle mass.[4] You want to maintain lean muscle for strength and functionality, but you should also note that muscle burns more calories than fat. In order to remain healthy, muscle tissue requires a number of metabolic "housekeeping" processes[5] that aren't necessary for the upkeep of fat. Those metabolic processes require energy, and energy is calories. If you don't use a muscle for an extended period of time, your body, being the efficient organism that it is, says, "Hey, we aren't using this stuff; let's get rid of it so we don't have to spend all of these calories maintaining it." So you can see how strength training can play a key role in weight loss and weight maintenance, not to mention that it's nice not to get weaker as you get older. Finally, strength training offers the added benefit of making you look much better once you do lose the fat. We would all prefer to be thin *and* toned, wouldn't we?

This is the time when you should really consider hiring a trainer, even just for one or two sessions, to work up a safe and effective program for you. There are so many different exercises and types of strength-training equipment available, it would take a lot of research on your part to figure out which might be the best for you. Add to that the dilemma of how much weight you should be lifting for how many sets and repetitions, and you can see where a novice could get overwhelmed. Beware of online forums, as they tend to be geared toward very experienced weight lifters. Getting your strength-training advice from a body-building website would be a little bit like me trying to learn how to fly an airplane by watching YouTube videos of fighter pilots.

Some gyms have exercise classes that incorporate a strength or calisthenic component. This can be a great free or low-cost way for you to get started. Just be sure to let the instructor know before your first class that you're a beginner, and tell him or her about any past injuries, current limitations, or health conditions you have so they can recommend any necessary modifications for you.

Regardless of what type of strength-training regimen you choose to follow, you should aim to do two or three strength workouts per week, on nonconsecutive days. An effective total body circuit can be completed twice through in about 30 minutes, including the warm-up.

## Using Exercise to Feel Younger

The other areas of fitness that you should not neglect include flexibility, posture, balance, and agility. These are the often-overlooked areas that have the potential to make your life so much better. Most people skip these forms of exercise because they offer little in the way of caloric expenditure, but I consider them to be preventative maintenance for my body and perform at least a few minutes of them almost every single day.

Many of our aches and pains are due to postural deficiencies from years of sitting at desks and bending our heads over books and computer screens. If we do stand, we normally do it badly, shifting our weight onto one leg or the other, slouching, sticking our bellies out over our toes. Years and years of this take a huge toll on our musculoskeletal system, causing back pain, neck pain, joint stiffness, and headaches. The only way to counter these negative side effects is to train the musculoskeletal system back into proper alignment, and of course, then to practice proper posture and alignment thereafter. Yoga, Pilates, tai chi, qigong, and some mild martial art forms place a huge emphasis on proper body alignment. They also incorporate a good mix of flexibility, balance, and agility training as well. At the bare minimum, you should do a 5- or 10-minute routine at the end of every cardio workout that incorporates stretching all of the major muscle groups, realigning your posture, and improving your balance and agility. Ask your trainer to show you which stretches to do and how to perform them properly.

## Variety Is the Spice of Exercise

For those of you who are shaking your heads no, thinking that you're happy to stick with your current exercise regimen, give me the chance to convince you otherwise.

There are two major benefits to changing up your exercise routine every couple of months. The first reason is to avoid injury. Sticking with the same workout program, doing the same exercises, on the same equipment, in the same order week after week can lead to an overuse or repetitive strain injury. These types of injuries are the result of imperfect form, body asymmetries, or just normal wear and tear. No matter how careful you are about form, none of us is perfect, and those slight imperfections in alignment, when done for hundreds or thousands of repetitions over a number of weeks, can lead to muscular or joint injury. The best way to avoid these injuries is to change what you're doing periodically so that your body isn't forced to move in the same exact pattern over time.

The second reason to change up your routine is to avoid those dreaded weight-loss plateaus. Remember, our bodies are highly adaptable, able to become proficient at doing a certain task or movement after just a few weeks. While this is desirable if you're trying to get good at a specific skill or movement (for sports, etc.), it's not desirable if you're trying to continue improving your physical condition. In order to do that, you'll need to force your body to keep adapting by placing new demands on it. This is true not only for muscular and cardiovascular fitness benefits but for burning calories as well. The less efficient your body is at performing a physical task, the more calories it expends in trying to complete that task. So once your body has adapted and an exercise starts to feel easier, it *really is* easier and you're not burning as many calories as you were when you first learned it. The difference in the calories burned is small, but over time, even very small calorie differences can add up. So do yourself a favor, and resist the temptation to stick with a routine once it's obviously become easy for you.

If you really love a particular activity and you can't bear to take a break from it (this happens a lot with runners or those who participate in a favorite sport), then you'll at least need to change the structure of those workouts. If you're running, for example, alternate the levels of intensity or the type of route (flat versus hilly, paved versus trail versus treadmill) on consecutive days. If basketball is your thing, don't play in competitive or pick-up games every day; spend at least two or three days a week working on conditioning, improving your shot, your ball-handling skills, or your vertical jump.

Those examples give you some idea of how you can do what you love nearly every day while minimizing your risk of injury, but the best course for both injury prevention and for avoiding plateaus is to alternate modes of exercise on consecutive days. A sample week might look something like this:

| Sunday | Dynamic Stretching and Agility | Fast, Short Walk |
|---|---|---|
| Monday | Aerobic Dance Class | |
| Tuesday | Strength Training | Hilly Walk |
| Wednesday | Yoga Class | |
| Thursday | Long Walk | Stretch and Balance |
| Friday | Dynamic Stretching and Agility | Fast, Short Walk |
| Saturday | Strength Training | |

In this example, the individual's preferred mode of exercise is walking, but he works in an aerobic dance class and his strength and flexibility workouts on the days in between his walks. He gets in some additional flexibility training and balance and agility work in the form of his warm-ups and cooldowns on his walk days. By not doing the same thing day after day, you'll avoid getting bored and you'll be more likely to up the intensity on one or two days of the week.

Another way to avoid injury and plateaus is by changing your program up entirely about every eight weeks. You can use the changing seasons to guide you, moving from walking or bicycling in the spring to swimming when it's hot in the middle of summer to hiking in the fall and cross-country skiing or snowshoeing in the winter. Because a season is typically more like twelve to sixteen weeks long, you'll want to make slight variations within your chosen activities around the eight-week point by choosing different routes, swimming different strokes, adding in interval training, or moving your workouts indoors to comparable gym-based equipment (like treadmills, stationary bicycles, and elliptical machines).

Your workout variety and progression is limited only by your imagination and your willingness to try new things or new ways of doing old things. Whatever your approach, try to avoid the tendency to get too comfortable doing the same workouts week after week.

## Duration or Intensity?

In Exercise 22, you started to step up your workouts a little bit. Maybe you decided to spend more time working out, or maybe you decided to work out a little harder. At this point, you should aim to exercise for at least 30 minutes most days of the week. The reason for this is that it's safer to increase duration before intensity, and you get some great fitness and health benefits from exercising longer. However, once you're consistently topping 30 minutes a day, it would be a good idea for you to turn your attention toward your effort level.

Just like duration, increasing intensity will help you get fitter and burn more calories. But intensity can also add a kind of variety to your workout program, where duration can often have the opposite effect. By simply doing what you've been doing for longer, you run the risk of getting bored, not only from day to day, but within the space of a single workout. However, by adding some jogging to a walk, doing some hill repeats on your bicycle, or practicing a more energy-demanding swimming stroke, you give your brain something new to learn or think about. Not only that, you'll be throwing your body a curve ball, making it adapt to something new, which can translate into favorable changes in metabolism.

## Hard Work Pays Off

If it sounds like I'm making the case for you to start upping your intensity, that's because I am. In the sections that follow, I'll tell you why. Exercise intensity can be a bit of a tricky area, though. How do you measure it? How do you know what's too easy and what's too hard? How do you know what's safe? Is it good to work out hard all the time? Fortunately, there are some reliable common-sense tips and tools that can help answer these questions.

## Finding the Right Effort Level

A great tool for determining the level of intensity that is right for you is the heart rate monitor. Cheap or expensive, most models will give you the basic information you need to objectively measure your effort level. For the first several weeks, generally healthy individuals should spend most of their training time in Zone 2, or at about 60 to 65 percent of maximum heart rate, which is the maximum rate your heart can beat for a sustained period of time. One way to get a rough estimate of your maximum heart rate (max HR) is to subtract your age from 220. The user guide that comes with your monitor might give you more detailed information on estimating max HR and explain the different zones, so take a look at that.

If you don't want to use a heart rate monitor, you can gauge intensity by using a rating of perceived exertion (RPE). This is a scale of 1 to 10, where a 1 is no effort at all (lying in bed) and 10 is maximum effort to the point of exhaustion. An RPE of 5 or 6 equals moderate effort. This is more subjective than using a heart rate monitor, but it's a better choice for individuals who take medication that affects their heart rate (such as beta blockers) or for those who don't want to be tied to a gadget every time they work out.

A third way you can measure your intensity is by using the talk test. When you first start exercising, start talking (the Pledge of Allegiance is a common thing I have clients recite). As soon as your rate of breathing increases to the point where it's just getting hard to complete full sentences, you know you're entering moderate-intensity territory.

These parameters I've mentioned—a heart rate around 65 percent of maximum, an RPE of 5 or 6, and the level where your breathing just becomes labored—are all what I call the "safe work zone." You're working at a level that is giving you a decent calorie burn and some aerobic benefits, and it's also a low-risk effort level for most individuals. If you've been working out at an intensity level below this up to now, you can start using this moderate zone as a target or goal to work up to.

## Intensity and Calorie Burn

If you're exercising at 50 percent max HR (or a 4 RPE) for every workout, then you're only getting a small calorie-burning benefit from exercise. Of course, if you're very deconditioned or have any health issues, then this is your mandatory starting place. (Check with your doctor to determine what is safe.) As a general rule, if you've been cleared by your doctor to exercise at a moderate level of intensity, then you should at least be breaking a light sweat, feel like your breathing is a bit more labored, and/or be hitting 60 percent of HR max. After a little while, you'll start feeling fit enough to push beyond those markers for short periods of time. This is when you can start incorporating intervals into your workouts, if you haven't been already.

Intervals were discussed in chapter 7, but here's a quick recap: they are short periods of hard effort followed by a recovery period of low or moderate effort. In the beginning, you should make the hard portion of your intervals very short, 20 or 30 seconds, and your recovery intervals at least twice as long. You can progress by either adding more intervals within the workout or by increasing the "work" period and decreasing the "recovery" period. Here are a couple of examples that illustrate those two progression options.

## Interval Workout (Total Duration, 30 Minutes)

- Warm up for 5 minutes, progressing from an easy to a moderate pace
- Increase speed/resistance/incline for 30 seconds
- Return to easy or moderate effort level for 2 minutes
- Repeat 4 times, for a total of 5 intervals
- Continue at moderate intensity for 8 minutes
- Cool down for 5 minutes

## Progression One (Total Duration, 30 Minutes)

- Warm up for 5 minutes, progressing from an easy to a moderate pace
- Increase speed/resistance/incline for 45 seconds
- Return to easy or moderate effort level for 90 seconds
- Repeat 4 times, for a total of 5 intervals
- Continue at moderate intensity for 9 minutes
- Cool down for 5 minutes

## Progression Two (Total Duration, 30 Minutes)

- Warm up for 5 minutes, progressing from an easy to a moderate pace
- Increase speed/resistance/incline for 30 seconds
- Return to easy or moderate effort level for 2 minutes
- Repeat 7 times, for a total of 8 intervals
- Cool down for 5 minutes

Once you've introduced some higher-intensity bouts into your workouts, you should start seeing bigger improvements in your aerobic fitness. The good news is that as you get fitter, you're able to burn more calories at the same *effort level* because you can go a bit faster or handle a slightly steeper incline or a higher resistance level. At this point, don't be tempted to keep your workout parameters the same, patting yourself on the back because it's so much easier now than it used to be. That's a great sign that you're fitter, but you should also recognize it as a sign that your body has adapted to those previous work levels. Remember that as your body adapts, it becomes more efficient, which means it is burning slightly *fewer* calories to perform the exact same workout than it was before.

If you hate the thought of exercising harder, you do have the option of keeping intensity the same but exercising longer. Note, however, that a "long" workout should be at least 45 minutes, and more than an hour is desirable. Remember too that between the variables of intensity and time, intensity has a bigger impact on your rate of calorie burn. This is because your *net* calorie burn is much greater at higher effort levels than at lower ones.

Here's an example that illustrates this: Say you're going to travel one mile on foot, and let's pretend you weigh 150 pounds. You decide to walk that mile at a good moderate pace of 3.5 miles per hour. It takes you 17.5 minutes and you burn about 77 calories doing it. Oh, but if you had been sitting on the couch for 17.5 minutes, you would have burned about 21 calories anyway, so your *net* calorie burn for walking one mile at 3.5 mph is 56 calories.

Now let's say you decide to jog that same mile at a moderate pace of 5.0 mph. It only takes you 12 minutes to cover the distance, but you burn 124 calories. During those 12 minutes, if you had been sitting on the couch, you would have burned 14 calories anyway, so your net calorie burn for jogging one mile at 5.0 mph is 110 calories.

There's already a pretty big difference in *gross* calories between walking and jogging that mile (61 percent), but the difference in *net* calories (56 walking and 110 jogging) is a whopping 97 percent increase!

There's one more piece to the calorie-burning puzzle you need to consider. In the last chapter, I told you that as you lose weight, your body burns fewer calories than it used to. This means that if you exercise when you're at your heaviest, your weight is actually working to your advantage. For heavy individuals, virtually any type of movement done for a stretch of 30 minutes or more will burn a significant number of calories. A 185-pound person who goes bowling for an hour will burn about 265 calories. The same person would expend 465 calories playing a 90-minute round of golf. A 30-minute walk at a brisk 3.5 mph would burn 155 calories, and if she is fit enough to jog at a 5.0 mph pace for those same 30 minutes, she'll burn 355 calories. However, after she's lost 30 pounds, her 155-pound self would burn around 15 percent fewer calories doing the exact same activities.[6]

These examples illustrate how the combination of intensity and duration can determine the caloric benefit of any given activity at a specific body weight. When you also factor in the *F* of *daily* frequency, you can see what a big effect activity can have on your weight-loss efforts. Just know that as you continue losing weight, you'll have to work a little harder and a little longer to keep realizing those benefits. So kick things up a notch, and delight in the fact that you're fitter now than you were just a few weeks ago. That's how positive change happens—steadily and progressively.

## Intensity—It's Not Just for Cardio

Up to now, I've been focusing on cardiovascular exercise, but it's possible and desirable to add intensity to your strength-training workouts as well. As with aerobic exercise, it's safer to first increase the strength-training equivalent of duration—the number of sets you do for each exercise. When you get started, you might only do one set of each exercise in your circuit while your muscles are getting used to the new demands you're placing on them. But as soon as you stop feeling soreness as a result of your strength workouts, you can increase the number of sets to two. Most people find that doing the exercises as a circuit twice through (do one set of each exercise in your routine, then repeat the whole thing when you get to the end) is a little less fatiguing than doing two sets of each exercise back-to-back before moving on to the next exercise in the circuit. (Back-to-back sets require a rest of at least 30 seconds between sets.)

Once you can comfortably complete your circuit twice through, the next progression is to either increase the number of repetitions you perform per set, or increase the amount of weight you're lifting for each exercise. If you increase the weight, you shouldn't raise it by more than 10 percent. If you're working with lighter weights and the next available weight is more than 10 percent heavier, then increase the number of repetitions first. Your trainer can tell you where you should be starting in terms of weight, repetitions, and sets, but as a general rule, you'll want to begin with a weight that you can lift *with perfect form* between 12 and 15 times for one set. If you are progressing by increasing repetitions, then you should work your way up to 20 repetitions before increasing the weight. If you're keen to pile on more weight right away, you should drop your repetitions down to the low end of that range (or even lower—somewhere between 10 and 12 repetitions) and gradually work your way back up to 15 reps or more before you add more weight again. Because there are so many variables at play with strength training, it really is a good idea to have a session or two with a certified professional first.

You should aim for progress in the areas of flexibility, balance, and agility as well. You can move on to more advanced yoga classes, strive to stretch a little farther for a little longer, and utilize devices that will really challenge your balance and agility, like balance pods, stability balls, and agility ladders.

While this information was not intended as an all-encompassing exercise guide for you, I hope it has helped to answer some of your questions and given you an idea of how many different options are out there and what the basic structure of a well-balanced exercise program looks like.

## Preventing Exercise Lapses

While it can be fairly simple to institute gradual changes in diet by substituting healthier options for less healthy ones, in the case of exercise you're adding something new that you weren't previously doing. This can make the habit of exercise a tough one to develop and an easy one to let slip away over time.

The best way to prevent that from happening is to remind yourself daily why it's so important and to set up an environment that maximizes your probability of success. Tell yourself every day that you are changing from the person you used to be into the person you want to be. You're a fit, active individual now, and exercise is one of the main elements of that new lifestyle. Think or say to yourself and others, "I'm a runner," or "I'm getting strong and lean," or "I'm going to be the fittest fifty-year-old I know."

*Tie your identity to your new lifestyle in as many ways as possible,*
*and don't stop reinforcing that belief in yourself.*

Once you *know* that you're an active person, the activity follows naturally. Why are you waking up at 5:00 a.m. to go for a jog? Because that's what runners do, and you're a runner. Why are you dragging yourself out of bed on a Sunday morning to go to the gym? Because exercise is the one constant in your life that you don't compromise on. You should create similar scripts for your chosen activities.

Another tip is to set yourself up for success rather than sabotage your best intentions by *minding the details.* Always have those workout clothes ready to go. Set two alarms to get up on time in the morning if that's when you work out. Have an alternate, inclement weather plan if your next workout is supposed to be outdoors. Make an exercise date with a friend or group of friends that you don't dare break. Do some research online when you have a few minutes and find new and interesting walking, hiking, or cycling trails in your area. Spending a little time thinking through possible obstacles to make sure your exercise sessions actually happen will pay huge dividends.

Keeping yourself motivated and ready to go and having a formal plan or schedule for your workouts will do so much to help you succeed.

Once you've learned these two supporting skills, it will be almost like your workouts are on autopilot. Then the only thing you need to deal with is your internal antagonist and all of the excuses he or she will try to come up with.

When that alarm goes off early in the morning, it's tempting to tell yourself that you'll make up your workout later in the day. If one of your kids comes home from school sick, it seems reasonable to decide that your afternoon workout won't happen. If your boss hands you a new project late in the day with a tight deadline, your evening spinning class at the gym seems doomed. And deep down, there may be a part of you secretly rejoicing because now you have a bona fide excuse to skip the workout you were dreading.

These are the times that will test your commitment, and how you respond to them will ultimately determine your success. I can't stress enough how important it is for you *not to let the normal drama of your life constitute an emergency.* You *should* skip your workouts in cases of true emergencies. But emergencies are things that happen once or twice a year. Accidents, the death or hospitalization of a close friend or family member, your own serious or prolonged illness, major plumbing catastrophes, tornadoes and hurricanes—*these* things are emergencies. Your boss's imagined urgency about a work project that will likely sit on his desk going nowhere for two days after you submit it is not an emergency. Nor is your child's unexpected illness. And certainly not the fact that you didn't get quite as much sleep as you'd wanted. These things are all just a part of your daily life, which now prioritizes exercise.

You'll have to suck it up and be tired that day or sneak in a nap later if possible. You'll have to resort to your planned (and practiced!) home workout while you care for your sick child. And if that work project really can't be delayed, you'll have to skip the spinning class and opt for a 30-minute brisk walk instead. It will clear your head and give you a much-needed break, leaving you rejuvenated and reenergized to finish the work project.

*The biggest difference between those who will succeed*
*and those who will not is the priority that healthy lifestyle habits take*
*relative to the other demands of daily life.*

So again, you have to ask yourself, "How important is this to me?" And if you say that it's very important, then you have to act like it's very important. If you find yourself regularly subordinating your workouts to things like working too many hours, running your kids around to different activities, caring for family members, or just because of a more ambiguous feeling of "busy-ness" or "stress," then you have not made your health a true priority. It is true that you have to do your work, your kids need to get to their activities, and family members will need to be cared for. And perhaps you are the person all of that falls to. But you're not a helpless victim of circumstance; you *must* choose to honor your commitments to your health first, and figure out how to accomplish the rest *afterward*. It's the only way this is going to work. If you're saying to yourself, "But I just can't do that right now," then I'm afraid you're right.

## The Other 930 Minutes of the Day

In the calorie-expenditure equation, exercise is the piece that you have the most control over, so it tends to get most (or often all) of the attention. But if you're only exercising for an average of 30 minutes a day, what about the other 930 minutes when you're awake but not exercising?

Physical activity can account for between 10 and 20 percent of our daily calorie expenditure. For those who exercise regularly, it's closer to 20 percent, which is twice as good as 10 percent, but that still leaves the other 80 percent. A few calories are burned through the digestion of food and regulation of body temperature, but it's normally a very small percentage. Of the calories expended every day, 60 to 70 percent are burned when you're not exercising—sitting at your desk at work or on the couch at home, walking to the fridge or the bathroom, when you're sleeping even. The body is using energy all the time in order to keep itself running smoothly. But what if you changed the nature of what you were doing for more of those 15.5 hours when you're awake but not working out? A time period that large could potentially deliver some pretty big payoffs.

An acronym has been coined to describe what I'm talking about here; it's called NEAT: Non-Exercise Activity Thermogenesis. NEAT consists of *any movement* you engage in during the day that is not part of your planned exercise. Walking up the stairs instead of taking the elevator; working at a stand-up workstation rather than at a traditional desk; parking farther from the store or your home or your work; simply performing a few "chair squats" at your desk every hour (stand up, sit down, stand up, sit down, stand up, sit down, done); spending family time after dinner walking around the neighborhood or playing catch in the yard rather than watching TV— these are all examples of how you can work more NEAT into your day.

You can see that by changing a few habits throughout your day—without investing a whole lot of time or effort into any one of them—you could burn a significant number of extra calories. Increasing NEAT by just 30 to 100 calories per day would result in between three and ten additional pounds lost per year. Imagine if, for the past ten years, you had been *losing* three to ten pounds each year rather than *gaining* them. Physically, you would be quite a different person!

So give NEAT some attention. Right now think through your typical day and jot down a list of areas where and when you could add small bouts of extra movement. Keep the list handy for a week or so to remind yourself, and before you know it, this "free" calorie burn will be second nature.

## Chapter Eleven

# YOU ARE HOW YOU EAT

In the same way that chapter 10 looked more closely at exercise, this is where we'll go deeper into diet. Depending on a number of factors, your transition to healthier eating may be fairly easy, or you might be ready to throw in the towel. For those of you who are struggling, what follows are some tips and suggestions designed to help you tackle this tough component of your new lifestyle.

## Change Your Relationship with Food

Whether you think you do or not, you have a relationship with the food you eat. Maybe you don't think about it much at all and just grab whatever is close at hand when it's convenient or when you're "starving." Maybe you think about it all the time, watching the clock, using your next snack break as a reward or an escape from a job or personal situation that's causing you stress or boredom. Maybe you're the typical lifelong dieter, carefully counting calories or carbs all day long, only to run out of willpower at the end of the day as you dive shamefully into a package of cookies or a pint of ice cream. However, most likely you have not carefully planned your meals to ensure that each one will supply the nutrients and energy needed to fuel your body's functions. You may not view food as fuel at all, and most of you have probably never thought of it as preventive or restorative medicine. To you, food is fun, it's tasty, and it's your enemy. You love it because it fills so many needs in your life, and you hate it because it has led to your current overweight condition.

Before you can begin to change the behaviors involving what actually goes into your mouth, you'll need to change the behaviors going on inside your head. Your attitude toward food—the way you think about it, depend on it, love it or fear it—determines what you will do with it. If you want to transform yourself into a thin, fit, healthy person, then

*Food must cease to be an emotional crutch or an item of convenience, and it must become a source of fuel and medicine instead.*

## Eat to Live

Of course food will still be a source of pleasure, and it will play a significant role in your social interactions, but more than any of those things, you need to learn the true purpose of the food and drink you put into your body: It is necessary to run and regulate your biological systems, and it supplies you with the energy to survive and thrive. It affects your immune system, your mood, your digestion, your energy levels, the production of your hormones, the regeneration of your cell tissue, how clearly you think, how well you sleep, and even your sexual performance.[1] The very important thing for you to realize is that food can affect all of these things in either positive or negative ways.

Unfortunately, the kind of food you've probably been eating does not promote health in any of these areas. Health-promoting, energy-fueling food doesn't come in a box or bag, or in 12-inch or 16-inch sizes with extra pepperoni. It doesn't come with a side of fries or a 32-ounce cola. It's not breaded or fried, and it doesn't have frosting on top. You can't cook it in a microwave or suck it through a straw. Good food is the stuff that was growing on a stalk or stem yesterday. It was recently wandering around a spacious, well-kept, grassy field or swimming freely in the ocean or a mountain stream. If it has been lightly processed, you can still tell what it started out as when you look at it. It hasn't been bleached or boiled or refined or transformed into a much different physical state than it was originally. The food that will fuel your body, keep you well, and actually halt, reverse, or heal your maladies is *whole food*. The closer your food is to the state it was in when it was alive or growing, the more powerful its benefits will be. So freshness is key, where it comes from is very important, and the method of preparation is essential. Beyond that, you have quite a bit of leeway with *what* you actually eat.

## "But I Don't Like That Stuff!"

I hear this a lot from clients when I have the whole food talk with them. My response is always the same: we're all capable of learning to like new foods. Studies on the human sense of taste have shown that it absolutely is possible for a person's palate to change as it is subjected to different tastes,[2] and it doesn't even take a very long time to happen. The European Food Information Council reports that while young children usually need to try a new food five to ten times before developing a taste for it, adults can more easily overcome their fear of new foods.[3] And here's some news: you might not actually dislike many of those healthy foods; you only *think* you dislike them. Humans have the tendency to rely heavily on memory, and we often assume that our tastes as adults are the same as they were when we were children or adolescents. But the truth is, our taste buds evolve with our biological development,[4] so it's possible that you might like a whole different range of foods now if you only expose yourself to them. Likewise, if you stop exposing yourself to other tastes (heavy doses of salt or sweetener, for example), you can pretty quickly lose the taste for those flavors.

## Welcome to Your New Mouth

The key to learning to like new foods is that you have to keep an open mind and a positive attitude when trying them. Don't let memory or assumptions color your current experience. If you tell yourself, "I'm going to hate this!" then you will. But if you say instead, "I didn't used to like this, but I might now," and after trying it, think, "I don't like this today, but I might like it tomorrow," you're doing two important things: you're being honest, rather than trying to trick yourself (which won't work), and you're giving yourself the chance to evolve at a later date.

Here are some practical tips that can help you reeducate your palate so you enjoy healthy foods.

### Try Different Methods of Preparation

I can eat broccoli raw, but I don't like it much. Steaming or boiling it makes it marginally better. If it's sautéed in a smidge of olive oil with a little red onion and thyme, I like it quite a bit more. But if I toss it with a little olive oil, red onion, and thyme and then roast it for 15 minutes in a 350-degree oven, I'll eat the whole pan in one sitting. As long as you're keeping the preparation methods and accompaniments in line with your overall dietary plan (i.e., no deep-frying, no cream-based or cheese sauces, etc.), you can feel free to cook healthy food any way you want. So don't be afraid to experiment and get creative, and if something is really awful, don't get discouraged; just move on and try something else. I once tried adding raw broccoli to my mid-morning smoothie. Yep, just once.

### Enlist Your Other Senses

Lending even more credibility to the idea that your tastes are not hard-wired, scientists have found that the color of a food can profoundly affect a person's impression of its taste.[5] I find this to be true for myself in the case of beets. I don't care at all for the purple variety, but I rather like the golden ones, and I'm pretty sure that if blindfolded, they would both taste the same to me. Another interesting study even found that music can have an effect on how yummy a person judges their food to be.[6] The researchers found that higher-pitched music tended to bring out the sweetness in foods, while lower-pitched pieces brought out the bitterness. So why not listen to a nice, light aria the next time you're giving kale a try?

### Think Outside the Box

It doesn't take a large amount of oil, acid, or seasoning to turn something blah into something grand. The right combination of textures and flavors makes all the difference. Get creative and find flavor combinations that you like. Don't limit yourself to the typical recipes for certain foods. Seek out things that sound different, interesting, and maybe even crazy. Try Moroccan spices in your mashed sweet potatoes; mix homemade salsa with black beans and wrap it in lettuce for a super-lean burrito; sweeten your steel-cut oats with a little molasses and pumpkin pie spice for "gingerbread oatmeal"; spread a tablespoon of low-fat cream cheese on a graham cracker and top it with fresh sliced strawberries—you won't believe it's not cheesecake! My favorite side dish for any meal is peeled and diced squash tossed with a teaspoon of olive oil, a tablespoon of soy sauce, and a sprinkling of a seaweed-sesame seed mixture known as furikake, baked at 350 degrees for 20 minutes. Taking stock of what you have on hand several times a week will not only spark ideas for combinations you can try, but it will also help you finish food before it goes bad, saving you a little money in the process.

### Seek Out a Variety of Recipes

There are some great food apps and websites that allow you to search for recipes by ingredient. Plug in the name of the food you're trying to learn to like and browse the many listings you're sure to get. Then pick two or three *healthy* recipes that you're willing to try. This is a good way to find new flavor combinations, and it's also a good way to hone your cooking skills.

## Speaking of Cooking Skills . . .

What—you don't cook?! "No time." "I hate it!" "I never learned how." "I'm horrible at it!" Well, this is a likely contributor to your current condition, and it's one of the few *mandatory* behaviors you'll need to implement. I don't expect you to cook every meal you eat from scratch, but your new fit-and-thin lifestyle requires that you are comfortable in the kitchen.

If you don't cook much (or at all), you should aim to increase the number of meals you prepare each week by one or two. If you have a willing spouse or housemate, then congratulations, you're off the hook, though it's still a good idea to have a working knowledge of basic healthy cooking skills.

There are many books, blogs, and websites with recipes and meal plans that go hand in hand with your chosen diet. Some of the better ones will have an introductory section that discusses healthy cooking methods and ingredients you may not be familiar with. Take a little time to find one or two solid resources that are easy to follow.

Start small with simple dishes that will taste good and require few steps and simple meal timing. These are your one-pot meals: soups, stews, whole-grain salads, stir-fries, and sautés. While they might be a little time-consuming with chopping and measuring requirements, clean-up will be minimal and you'll be rewarded with six to ten servings of delicious, healthy food to get you through the next few days.

Another easy way to instantly boost the quality of your diet is to add a big salad to every lunch and dinner. That way, even when you don't have time to cook a whole meal and you're forced to eat something packaged or from a restaurant, you'll still get a healthy dose of fresh vegetables that provide nourishment and fill you up. Just watch out for salad dressing, meat, and cheese—putting these on top of your fresh veggies can turn a 200-calorie power meal into an 800-calorie fat bomb. The best dressings are the simplest: mix together a tiny bit of oil (olive or flax are good) with an equal amount of acid (vinegar, lemon or lime juice) and a little sweetener (I like honey or maple syrup, depending on what I'm putting in my salad, what type of vinegar I'm using, etc.). My favorite dressing isn't even a dressing! I mash up one-quarter of a ripe avocado and squeeze half a lemon onto the salad, season with a little salt and pepper, then mix it all together with my fingertips to coat the whole salad. Try it sometime—it's amazing!

Apart from salads and one-pot meals, you can make things really simple for yourself by using the plate method. Mix and match foods from the following general categories to fill your plate *every time you eat*: Vegetables, 30 percent; Fruit, 15 percent; Lean Protein, 25 percent; Whole Grains, 25 percent. You can see a visual representation of this plate at http://www.hsph.harvard.edu/nutritionsource.

## Change the Way You Cook the Foods You Already Eat

If you already cook at home a little, then you might not need to drastically change *what* you eat. It's possible to cut a ton of fat and calories just by changing the *way* your food is prepared. By examining your latest seven days' worth of food logging, you should be able to see whether you can prepare your food in a healthier way. This assumes you have been diligent with your food logging (counting calories for oil used in cooking; seeds, nuts, or cheese used for garnish, etc.).

Here's a general hierarchy of nutritive value among various methods of preparation for nearly all foods, from most to least healthy:

| Plant-Based Foods | Animal Products |
| --- | --- |
| Raw | Grilled* |
| Blended, Pureed, or Juiced** | Poached or Boiled |
| Steamed or Baked | Roasted or Baked |
| Boiled | Lightly Seared, Browned, or Braised |
| Lightly Sautéed or Braised | Pan-Fried |
| Fried | Deep-Fried |
| Breaded and Deep-Fried | Highly Processed and/or Cured |

\* While grilling meats is generally considered to be a low-calorie method of preparation, some studies have shown that grilling meat over a high heat can introduce potentially carcinogenic compounds.[7] Grilling slowly over lower, indirect heat is a safer way to prepare meat.

\*\* Juicing fruits and vegetables retains around 90 to 95 percent of the calories and nutrients of the whole food, but loses nearly 100 percent of the fiber. This can mean lots of calories without much satiety. I would recommend a good blender over a juicer any day, and you should limit consumption of blended drinks to one per day.

## Some Other Tips You Can Try

Here are some other common tips and tricks that might help you make the transition to healthier eating habits. Some of them have been widely covered by the mainstream media or are included in popular weight-loss programs, so you might have heard about them and tried them already, but they're all based on sound approaches and they bear mentioning again here.

Most likely, not all of these tips will work for you. Maybe only one of them will. You might even have to *modify* one or two to get them to work for you. But when you find something that does work, recognize it, celebrate it, and stick with it!

### Do a Pantry Inventory and Purge

If you're going to do this thing, you might as well get serious about it. How many times have you planned to turn over a new leaf and start eating healthy *just as soon as you eat up all the bad stuff in the house*? Does that day ever arrive? It never has in my house. Around here, the only way we succeed in revamping what we eat is by purging our supplies of everything on the "Do Not Eat" (DNE) list.

My spouse and I sit down together and make an agreed-upon list of which items we'll no longer be buying and eating. Every once in a while there will be an item that one of us may not want to give up but the other can't have it around, so we keep the "forbidden" food at the person's workplace or in a secret hiding spot where only the one who wants to eat it can access it. (This is not recommended for perishable items!)

Once the list is made, we then purge our pantry shelves, cupboards, refrigerator, and freezer of the DNE items. Most of the stuff we give away to neighbors or family members, but a good deal of leftovers or partially used packaged items just get thrown out.

After we've gotten rid of the bad foodstuffs, we thoroughly clean and organize the kitchen to make way for all of the healthy provisions we will restock the shelves with. While we're doing this, we compose a list of staple items to buy and keep on hand. Then we sit down together and plan our first week's worth of meals and write out a grocery list.

Doing this activity is a little time-consuming—about two to four hours total, depending on how much stuff we have on hand to dispense with—but it is a very important part of our process. It represents the seriousness of our commitment to a renewed way of healthy eating, and it is symbolic of the entire process we are changing—out with the old, in with the new! We do this one or two times per year, whenever one of us notices that we are straying from our "Food Is Medicine" orthodoxy.

## Match Your Dollars to Your Calories

A handy mantra to remember is this: willpower happens at the grocery store and not at home. Once you've brought something into your house, it will be eaten! So what can you do to make better choices when you're staring at those tempting end-cap offers at the grocery store? Here are a couple of tricks or "rules" you can follow to help you stick to the list and bring home only what you really should be eating.

First, identify your allowable daily "discretionary" or "empty" calorie total. These are calories from unhealthy beverages, desserts, fried foods, etc. A good rule of thumb is to limit these calories to around 10 to 15 percent of your daily total. Now take a look at your meal plan and resulting shopping list for the week. It should be easy for you to identify those items that fall into the empty-calorie category. These are things like added oils or sauces, high-fat dairy, any type of sugar, packaged snacks, caloric beverages (other than low-fat dairy or plant-based milks), etc. If there are more than one or two of these items on your list, you should really think about that.

What you'll do next is curb the amount of empty-calorie food you eat by tying it directly to dollars. Plug your allowed empty-calorie percentage (10 percent or so) into your grocery bill. If you're spending $70 for the next few days' worth of food, then you should be spending no more than $7 on less healthy items. If you really want to cut down how much junk you're buying, take a ten-dollar bill to the grocery store with you every time you go and have the cashier ring your food in two separate transactions—pay for your healthy food items on a debit or charge card, but make yourself pay cash for things you'd be better off skipping. You can follow this same "cash-for-junk" principle at restaurants too. The hassle of taking this extra step is likely to make you skip the junk food altogether.

## Stop Buying in Bulk

Aren't those big-box "club" stores great? They save you so much money, right? Wrong! Strong evidence says that the average wholesale club shopper spends more annually than they would if they just shopped at regular stores.[8] What's much worse, though, is the disastrous effect bulk buying can have on your dietary efforts.

The whole mentality of "stocking up" ties in to emotional and psychological needs that are likely contributors to your overweight condition. Think about why you shop this way. Are you worried that you'll run out of something? Do you feel it's more convenient to buy in bulk? Do you think it's cheaper? Well, you won't, it's not, and it's not.

"Running out" of food is the new way you *want* to plan, shop, and eat. Whole foods won't last on a shelf for a month, so don't buy a month's worth. Packaged food will, but that's the kind of stuff you're trying to phase out of your diet.

Stocking up on huge packages of stuff is only more convenient if you have the space to store it and about two hours to spend when you get home from the store opening packages and putting things away in two or three different locations—the place where you'll use it now, the one where you can get to it later, and (mercy!) that dark spot under the stairs where everything else goes. If you buy large amounts of food that isn't loaded with preservatives, then you'll have to divide that up and store most of it away in a refrigerator or freezer, which means that you'll probably have to buy a second or third refrigerator and/or freezer.

So quit hoarding cases of soda and boxes of candy bars and crates of peaches from Colorado. Buy what you need *this week*, based on your carefully planned list. Your waistline will be thinner and your wallet will be fatter.

# Challenge Yourself

Once you've brought the right kind of food home from the grocery store, how can you go about actually getting it into your mouth? There are a couple of fun challenges you can involve the whole family in that will automatically boost the health quotient of your diet.

## *Rainbow Challenge*

This is a challenge I started running periodically on my blog a few years ago. For one whole week (or longer, if you like) make it a goal to eat one serving of fruit or vegetable every day from every color of the rainbow: red, orange, yellow, green, purple/blue (or purple *and* blue for extra credit). Of course, your choices need to be healthfully prepared, but apart from that, there are no rules. A serving equals 1/2 cup of fruit (or one small apple, orange, pear, banana, etc.) and 3/4 cup of vegetable (or 2 cups, in the case of leafy greens). You can pick the color on the inside (such as green for kiwi) or the color on the outside (such as purple for eggplant).

This is an easy one to get kids involved with, because they love to roam the produce aisles picking out the colors of the rainbow. Scoring goes like this: 1 point per day for getting all the colors; 1 extra-credit point for each day that you log a purple and a blue (in addition to all other colors); 1 extra-credit point for each day where at least three of your servings were from vegetables. A one-week score of 10 or more puts you in the "Winner" category, 15 or more makes you a "Champ," and a score of 20 or 21 gives you "Leprechaun" status, because you've obviously found gold at the end of the rainbow!

### Whole-Grain Challenge

This challenge is not quite as much fun as the Rainbow Challenge, but it's potentially better for you. This challenge runs over the course of a month, and you are to pick a different whole grain to cook with each week. Try to really get creative with this one, choosing three or four different recipes featuring your grain of the week. Those who enjoy cooking and trying new things will love this challenge, and will likely gain a dozen or more great new recipes during the process. For those who are not as motivated, it will at least expose you to a few different new and healthy alternatives to rice and pasta. I haven't come up with a scoring scheme for this challenge (that's why it's not as much fun), but if you think of one, you can post it to my blog at www.wellcuratedlife .com/whole-grain-challenge/.

## Dish Size and Color Matter

Here's a funny old trick that has serious backing from some new studies. Over and over, weight-loss researchers have found that the size of the dish a person eats or drinks from directly correlates to how many calories are consumed during a meal.[9] What's more, perceptions of fullness among participants in one study were about the same, despite differences in calories consumed.[10] That means that eating your dinner off of a smaller plate not only will likely make you eat less than you otherwise would, but you'll probably feel just as full and satisfied as if you had eaten more food off of a bigger plate.

In addition to dish size, the color of your plate can also affect how much you eat. Studies have shown that if the color of your plate contrasts with the food you're serving, you're likely to eat less. In 1856, a Belgian scientist named Joseph Delboef discovered this principle, and in 2012, Drs. Brian Wansink and Koert van Ittersum confirmed it in a study that randomly served pasta with either marinara or Alfredo sauce on either red or white plates. Those who got the marinara on a white plate or the Alfredo on a red plate felt fuller and didn't eat as much as those who were offered the exact same portion size served on a sauce-matching plate. The researchers concluded that subjects perceived the portions served on contrasting plates to be larger.[11]

## Five More Tips for Healthier Eating

1. Only eat when you're sitting down at a dining table. Not in your car, at your desk, at your kids' sporting event, or standing over the kitchen sink.

2. When you eat, stop doing everything else. Pay attention to your food; savor it. Take a break from what you were doing and focus on this one activity.

3. Trade fast food for slow food. I'm not only talking about restaurants here. Stop eating microwavable entrées and packaged snacks. Cook your food and enjoy the whole process from start to finish. Snack on nuts in the shell, fruit with seeds or pits—things that will slow you down and force you to interact with the food rather than just shoving a handful of something into your mouth.

4. Drink water throughout the day. Don't wait until you're thirsty. Keep a refillable water bottle or a glass and filtered pitcher nearby and drink from it often. When you wake in the morning, drink at least 20 ounces of water before you ingest anything else. Always drink a full glass of water at mealtimes. Staying hydrated can help curb feelings of hunger.

5. Eat more often. Keep healthy snacks with you all of the time. Eat every two to three hours. Intentionally try to even out your calorie consumption across the day rather than getting a large percentage of your calories in the evening. This will keep your energy levels steady, will help curb cravings, and will make it easier to eat smaller portions of higher-calorie foods at mealtime. Snacks should be whole fruits or vegetables whenever possible, and should constitute no more than 10 percent of your daily calorie target per serving.

## Navigating the Dangerous Waters of Dining Out

Almost without exception, a meal out is less healthy than one made at home. Even "healthy" dishes served at "healthy" restaurants will nearly always contain more fat, salt, and sugar than the same meal you would make in your own kitchen. There are very few exceptions to this, so just assume that when you dine out you're getting more calories, fat, sodium, and sugar than you probably want. That's one reason why learning to cook at home is so important. Still, there are times when we all want or need to dine out, and some people can't avoid it because their jobs require them to frequently travel or entertain clients. Whatever your reasons for dining out are, there are a couple of things you can do to mitigate the damage.

### Restaurant Preplanning

First, you should view the menu of the restaurant online ahead of time. Nearly every restaurant has a website these days, and if it has a website, it will likely include a menu page. It's important for you to scan the menu and choose your meal before you arrive. Doing this in a setting other than the restaurant, away from the other people you'll be dining with, allows you to make a conscious, calculated choice based on your own dietary criteria rather than getting swept up in the group mentality, or being tempted by the aromas and ambiance of the restaurant.

Next, when you order your meal, ask the server if it's possible to get a lunch portion or if you can have half the meal boxed to go right from the start. I know this sounds like an extreme measure, and those of you who are shy won't want to do it, but remember that you are paying for this meal and for the service that comes along with it, so why not have it the way you want it? Having half the meal boxed up will keep you from eating the overly large portion that's likely to be served. If you're at a fine-dining establishment, the portions may not be as large, so you probably won't want to ask for a to-go box ahead of time. In this case, when your food arrives, after appreciating the lovely presentation of the dish, immediately parse out the portion you want to eat, and create visible space on your plate between that portion and the rest. Use that space as a virtual to-go box, and consider that food out of sight.

It's never a good idea to have an appetizer or dig into the bread basket before a meal, because somehow we've come to disregard these items—we don't think they "count" as part of the meal and so we're likely to eat them *as well as* the whole entrée when it arrives. So do yourself a favor and skip the bread, or the potato skins, or the calamari, and opt for a large, clean, lightly dressed salad instead.

### Mind Thy Drink!

Food is not the only caloric thing we consume, and I've already said that many people get a significant percentage of their daily calories from beverages of one sort or another. Whether it be creamy, sweetened coffee drinks, sugary sodas and juices, or alcohol, many beverages can contain upward of 200 calories for the portion normally consumed. Virtually all of those calories are empty ones, or worse, they are actually harmful to your health. The types of sweetener used in most coffee drinks and full-calorie sodas do more than just spike blood sugar. The ill effects of high-fructose corn syrup are well-documented in the scientific literature.[12] Similarly, alcohol, while potentially beneficial in very moderate quantities (1 to 2 ounces per day, maximum), is frequently consumed in much higher quantities, creating a host of negative health consequences. Some diet soft drinks can be a better choice, but only if consumed in moderation, as many of them still have amazingly high levels of sodium, and the long-term health effects of artificial sweeteners are not yet known. Additionally, studies have shown that regular drinkers of diet soda actually gain weight rather than lose weight—not as a direct result of the soda, but because they "make up" for those calories elsewhere in their diet.[13]

So what can a person do, other than drink plain old water? Well, there are some great calorie-free, sparkling water beverages (flavored only with a bit of real fruit juice and not artificially sweetened) on the market, and hot or iced herbal tea can be as comforting or refreshing as just about anything. But if you've really got the hankering for a cocktail, a glass of wine, a beer, or that irresistible coffee drink, then you'll have to learn to enjoy those things in extreme moderation. You'll also have to work them into your daily calorie allowance and, more importantly, into your daily *discretionary* calorie allowance. In many cases, that one coffee drink, beer, or cocktail will use up *all* of your empty calories for the day.

Hear what I am saying: Skipping lunch so you can hit the bar at happy hour will put you on the express train to weight-loss failure! But having a drink or two with friends in lieu of the dessert you had planned is okay *once in a while*. However, if you are of the opinion that things just aren't as much fun without the booze, then your issue is not with the calories, but with the alcohol itself, and you may want to explore whether you should seek help for this. The same is true of that six-pack-a-day soda habit, or the daily double mocha latte. If you feel that your happiness is closely tied to your regular daily drug of choice, then we're talking about a dependency, if not an addiction, and that is something beyond the scope of this book. It will be very difficult for you to successfully lose weight and keep it off if you have an addiction to sugar, alcohol, or caffeine. (I mention caffeine because many people don't drink their coffee black but add high-calorie cream and/or sugar.)

If dependency is not your issue, then on those occasions when you find yourself out with a crowd and surrounded by tempting beverages, at the very least implement the "every other" rule. If you're imbibing in alcoholic drinks or sodas at a party, be sure to make every other drink a full glass of water, tea, or sparkling water. This will keep you hydrated, keep you full, and slow down your rate of consumption of those empty-calorie beverages. Oh, and you'll thank me in the morning when you don't wake up with a splitting headache!

# Food Portion, Order, and Timing

Regardless of where you eat or how healthy your food choices are, if you struggle with portion control or overeating, then weight loss is bound to be difficult for you. While you may need to seek professional guidance depending on the severity of your issue, these next few tips can help many people limit how much food they take in at one sitting.

## Follow the Rule of Proportions

The Rule of Proportions says that with every meal, half of your plate should be made up of vegetables and/or fruits, with the remaining half being split between lean protein and whole grains. Often, for lunch or dinner, I'll meet the vegetable requirement with a big salad. Fruit should only factor in during breakfast or for snacks or dessert because it has many more calories and is much higher in sugar than vegetables are.

You can buy plates that are sectioned (think upscale church potluck plates or school lunch trays) and even color-coded, cueing you to place a small serving of protein here, a small serving of whole grains here, and a large serving of vegetables there. You can also buy bowls and glasses of a specific, premeasured size, or you can do what I do and eat out of glass food storage containers. This is especially effective for high-calorie dishes like pasta and whole-grain or bean salads. It can make food logging easy too—just fill up the dish and you'll know exactly what portion size you're eating.

## Everything in Good Order

Another way to avoid consuming too many calories per sitting is to fill up on low-calorie stuff first. Eating your serving of vegetables or fruits at the beginning of a meal will often result in consuming fewer total calories by the end of the meal. When those high-fiber foods hit your stomach, signals are sent to your brain telling it to slow down because you're filling up. It's a good idea to listen to your brain at that time and actually eat a little slower. That will give you the chance to decide that you're done before you've crammed in a couple hundred more calories.

## Drink Water Throughout the Meal

Regardless of what you're eating or what beverage you're pairing with your meal, you should have a full glass of water with your meal in addition to any juice, wine, beer, soda, etc., and you should drink your water glass empty before your other beverage (if you're having one) runs dry. This not only helps you feel fuller due to the bulk of the water in your stomach, but oftentimes our brains mistakenly perceive thirst as hunger, so satiating your thirst might tell your brain that you're done eating sooner.

### Dessert Last, or Not at All

Finally, if you're like me, you often crave a little something sweet right after a savory meal. But you'll probably find that if you wait about 15 minutes, that craving will usually go away. You can even distract yourself by getting up from the table and doing something active as soon as you've finished eating. My favorite post-dinner activity is a nice, leisurely walk around the block with the dogs, but more often than not it involves doing the dishes instead. In any case, removing yourself from the immediate eating environment can magically make your dessert cravings disappear.

### Mindfulness and Meal Timing

The timing of your meals and snacks throughout the day can be important. Going too long between meals or snacks can make your brain overproduce the hormones that signal hunger, causing you to gorge on whatever's put in front of you when you finally do eat.[14] Whether you prefer to eat three larger meals per day and no snacks, or three light meals and two or three small snacks, just remember to check in with yourself every few hours to see whether you're feeling hungry or experiencing a dip in energy. If you are, then grab a healthy snack—preferably some fresh veggies or fruit.

At night, it's important to eat dinner late enough to help prevent snacking before bedtime, but not so late that the digestion of your meal interferes with your sleep. I shoot for around 7:00 or 8:00, or about three hours before I go to bed, but this will vary depending on your schedule and any issues you might have with digestion and sleep.

## Physical Hunger vs. Emotional Want

For many, portion sizes are not a problem, or at least not the only problem. Some people engage in what is broadly labeled "emotional eating." In a nutshell, emotional eating happens when you're not really physically hungry, but you use food or beverage to fill some other need you falsely perceive as hunger. Virtually everyone does this on occasion, but for some, emotional eating is a habitual force that can become so severe it constitutes disordered eating. Chances are, you fall somewhere along the spectrum and not at either end of it, but if you often find yourself giving in to "cravings" for certain foods, or eating as the result of external stimuli (like TV commercials or coaxing from friends), then emotional eating may be a primary reason for why you are overweight now.

Your food log can help shine a light on this, especially if you've been utilizing the comment field, noting how you're feeling and why you're eating particular foods at particular times. If you suspect that a significant number of your daily calories are consumed when you're not really physically hungry, there are some actions you can take to help break out of those habits and to start listening to your body instead.

First, try this test: The next time you think you're hungry, imagine what you'd most like to eat. Probably, a specific food or flavor (sweet, salty, etc.) will jump to the front of your mind. Next, ask yourself if you could eat something entirely different right at that moment. Example: If you're craving something sweet—cookies, a sweet coffee drink or soda, pineapple or other sweet fruit, etc.—ask yourself if instead you could eat something like a carrot stick, a salad, or a grilled chicken breast. Then pay attention to what physically happens in your body when you shift your thoughts from cookies to a chicken breast. If you feel your hunger pass, or if you find yourself thinking, "No, that's not what I'm hungry for," then you aren't *really* hungry at all; you are experiencing a craving, and cravings are largely mental/emotional. If you are truly hungry, any type of food that you regularly eat should sound good to you. Then it's up to you to decide what to eat at that moment.

If you've done the above and established that you're not really hungry but you still want to eat something, try drinking 8 to 12 ounces of water. Your body might really be thirsty, but your brain is misperceiving your thirst as hunger.

If the water doesn't do the trick, try spending a few minutes writing down (or just mentally thinking about) why you might be craving this certain food. What's going on in your day right now? What external factors might be influencing you? Are you tired, stressed, nervous, or angry? Are you trying to put something undesirable off until later? Is someone in the next cubicle eating this thing? Did you just see a commercial on TV that triggered the craving? Chances are, if you can identify your trigger right there in the moment, you can overcome the craving.

Another way to overcome a craving is to use logic against it. At times, food cravings can seem insurmountable. We give them a life of their own, and they become powerful adversaries. But if you can step back and identify a craving for what it really is—a small, *passing* mental or emotional response to some learned trigger—then suddenly your chances of overcoming it seem much better than they did a moment earlier.

If the desire still persists, then you'll have to negotiate with yourself. You're experiencing a stubborn craving, and you have two choices for dealing with it: wait it out until it passes (and I promise you that it will), or give in to it. The result of each of those options should be clear to you. Now you can make a mindful, conscious decision about what you want to do, knowing what effect your decision will have on your weight-loss effort.

If you decide to wait it out, you can make it easier on yourself by using a positive distraction or two. If you're at work, chances are you have something you could be doing—dive in and do your best job. If you're not at work, or if you're able to take a break for a few minutes, take a short walk, get up and practice your posture exercises, do some stretches, or practice meditative breathing for a minute or two. By substituting something enjoyable or at least productive in place of the eating, you'll be giving yourself double benefits. You're not taking in a bunch of empty calories, and you're doing something else that's good for you.

Once you've practiced this response a few times, you'll find it increasingly easier to dismiss those familiar food cravings right when you first feel them. At times you will give in and eat when you're not truly hungry, but at least it will no longer be a mindless habit. Recognizing what you're doing in the moment is a key step to behavior change.

## Chapter Twelve

# LIKE IT OR NOT, YOU ARE IN CONTROL

**B**ehind the food you eat, the beverages you drink, and the exercises you do lies the one key thing that causes you to take the actions you take and behave the way you do: decisions.

If you're honest with yourself, you'll admit that every single thing you do from the time you wake up to the time you go to bed at night involves a decision that *you* make. In each instance, you have a choice, and it's how you choose to act time and again that begins to form your behaviors, your habits, and even what you've come to think of as your personality, or your "self." Admittedly, often there is really only one way to go with a decision because if you chose the other option the result would be disastrous—you "have to" go to work each day or you'll lose your job. You "have to" pick your child up from day care or he will be stuck there and social services will be called. You "have to" pay the electric bill or the lights will go out. So there are many decisions throughout the course of a day that, in essence, make themselves. Part of the trouble you had prior to starting this program was that you'd been applying this same autopilot framework to many of your *other* decisions. Now is the time to ask yourself whether that is still the case.

If you automatically eat X for breakfast every morning, that could be a problem. If you automatically pop open a beer or uncork a bottle of wine when you get home from work, that could be a problem. If you routinely skip your trip to the gym when traffic is bad, that could be a problem.

Some of these nondecisions are the result of habit or a lack of mindfulness, and some of them are the product of a convenient excuse you've made for yourself. In either case, each time you pass up the opportunity to make a conscious, well-thought-out decision, you move further away from reaching your goals.

Mastering behavior change begins with consciously making as many decisions as you possibly can every day. It requires you to be engaged in your life in a way you haven't been. It forces you to look at the options and the consequences of each choice, and then take deliberate action. This can be uncomfortable, because it rids you of your excuses or your blissful ignorance and forces you to acknowledge that *you are responsible for your life*. Suddenly, negative things don't "happen" to you but are revealed as owing, at least in part, to a choice you've made. This is the most powerful revelation you can come to: the fact that you control what you do each and every day.

Of course, you can't control others, and you shouldn't try to. You can't control many circumstances or conditions outside of your own very limited realm either. But you can control how you *react* to those other people, circumstances, and conditions, and in many cases, you can even control whether you're exposed to them at all.

Behavior change is hard. It forces you to confront difficult issues and ask yourself uncomfortable questions. You might find yourself wanting to skip over them and tell yourself they don't apply to you. I urge you to pause in those moments, be honest with yourself, and consciously make a decision. When you find yourself thinking, "I can't do that because of X," just really give it some thought and ask yourself how much control you truly have. I think you'll be surprised to find that once you change your usual way of thinking (or not thinking) about your attitudes and behaviors—once you force yourself to make those decisions—you'll start seeing progress where there were only roadblocks before.

## Are You Your Biggest Obstacle?

I've said already that excuses and guilt are both useless to this process, but you might be bringing something else into it that is not merely useless but toxic—your attitude. There are many ways to think about attitude and many ways to go about trying to change it, but none are more pertinent than what I call the Power of Perception.

Experts on stress management and happiness agree that the difference between those who are happiest and those who are miserable has little to do with external circumstances. Rather, it is *the way those circumstances are perceived* that determines how an individual will feel about his or her life. You might have heard about the study that found that one year after the event, individuals who won the lottery and individuals who tragically lost the use of their legs reported being equally happy.[1] Certainly the individual characteristics of these two groups' lives are very different. Happiness, then, apparently hinges much more on what we choose to focus on than it does on what we "have."

On a more personal level, you may often compare yourself to that friend you have whose life is magically perfect (you know the one): she has the job she loves, the house she always wanted, a great family; she's always going on fabulous trips, wears the latest fashions . . . yeah, *that* friend. How does your life compare to hers? Yours looks pretty cruddy, right? But now compare yourself to that other friend you have whose life is truly quite awful (you know the one): she lost her job, her health is poor, she's had a string of misfortunes, and she is really struggling just to get by. I'll bet your life looks pretty good in comparison.

We can do the same comparative exercise with just about everything in life. Things that we self-identify as "bad" or "stressful" are seldom as bad or as stressful as we work them up to be in our minds. If we step back and ask ourselves, "What's the real damage here?" or "What's the worst thing that can happen?" we will often find that the world, in fact, is not coming to an end.

You need look no further than those around you to find examples of how attitude can significantly affect happiness and success. Among your friends and acquaintances there are probably a few who have a lot to deal with in life and who do an incredible job of handling it all. These are the people who seem to have more hours in the day than the rest of us. They find time for exercise, eat healthfully, excel in the workplace, and make time for their families. Then there are others who cope quite poorly with the basket they've been handed, struggling just to get through the day, often complaining as they go. There are important lessons to learn from both groups.

First, you'll begin to see that your problems, or the demands being placed upon you, are not unique to you. There are a lot of people out there dealing with similar or worse situations than yours. Second, it allows you to pick and choose your role models from among the group who are doing extraordinarily well. Get to know them better, see what their tricks and habits are, and apply those tricks and habits to your own situations. Finally, it allows you to be grateful that you have it better than a lot of other people. It can be pretty motivating to realize, "I really have nothing to complain about. I am *able* to do this, so I should be *happy* to do it."

If you're able to change the way you view things, so that even on your worst days you can look around you and say, "This is pretty bad, but it's not bad enough to get the best of me. I can do this," then you will truly be in control and nothing will keep you from reaching your goals.

## Rally Your Supporters, Ditch Your Detractors

Maybe *your* attitude about this whole thing is just fine, and it's other people who are presenting the biggest challenges to your effort. Way back in Exercise 5 you told everyone important to you about your weight-loss effort. You also classified each person as either a Super Supporter, a Supporter, someone who was On the Fence, or a Detractor. No doubt, you probably were surprised by the reactions of a few people. From some, you might have gotten much more support than you had expected. Maybe your spouse or an older child offered to start cooking healthier meals. Maybe an old friend you'd lost touch with suggested that you reconnect and attend a fitness class together. Others may have decided to join you and try to lose some weight themselves. But you probably also got some negative reactions from one or two people you really thought you could count on.

I mentioned that might happen because those people somehow feel threatened by your new weight-loss effort. Maybe they fear that your relationship with them will change. Maybe they feel guilty because they know they should be making a weight-loss effort of their own. The reasons are unique to each individual, and there's nothing you can do about how another person feels about something. What you *can* control is your reaction to them.

Communicating effectively with your detractors is the only way to preserve that relationship without compromising your goals. Let them know that they are important to you, but that, for right now, losing weight is your top priority. Give them a list of reasons why you want to lose weight. Assure them that while some of your activities may change, your relationship with them can stay fundamentally the same. But be honest with them too—tell them that if you are successful, your life and you will be different than they are now. You'll enjoy doing different things; you probably won't frequent the same dining establishments; you won't be the person they can split the fried appetizer platter with anymore; you won't be spending as much time doing certain things because your new healthy habits will take a higher priority.

Then watch their response and ask yourself, "Does this person value me for who I am, or only for what I can offer them?" A true friend or loved one should recognize that what is important to you is also important to them. That doesn't mean this won't be a difficult process for you both, but it should mean that they ultimately will become a supporter rather than a detractor.

Remember that detractors can be people you like or even love. They just happen to also be the people who are impeding your progress by tempting you away from your healthy new behaviors. Hopefully, they will see how important this is to you and realize that they need to become supporters or at least stay out of your way. But there may be some who will simply continue putting their own interests ahead of yours, so you should be prepared for that possibility. If you think about it, it's actually a natural tendency—we all instinctively put our own interests first, right? The difference with detractors, though, is that they put their interests first *to your detriment*. They don't see (or won't see) that your health, even perhaps your life, is more important than their fun time.

When dealing with detractors, you'll need to be persistent, and a little creative. When you turn down an invitation from your friend to go out for ice cream or happy hour, don't just leave it at that—invite him or her to do an alternate activity with you. Suggest that you go to a movie or for a walk instead. Eventually your friend will either join you on your healthier outings (the best scenario), will stay your friend but respect that you no longer want to participate in unhealthy activities (an okay scenario), or will lose touch with you altogether. That last possibility is a sad one, but you need to be willing to make that decision and accept it if you are truly going to change your lifestyle and your life.

It's dangerous to think that you can go to the same places with the same people who are doing the same things you used to do and rely on your willpower to keep you from falling back into those old habits. Certainly you can occasionally go out with friends and indulge a little, or you can order the salad, grilled fish, and sparkling water while they live it up, but frequently putting yourself in those kinds of situations risks your long-term effort.

Spend your social-emotional time and energy where it counts most.

From this point forward, grab hold of those enthusiastic supporters and embrace them! Draw them close to you, nurture those relationships, and begin directing your social interactions toward your new lifestyle with those people in your closest circle and by your side. Bring to mind the picture of yourself in the future. What kinds of activities are you doing with friends and family? Hold that vision in your mind as you interact with your circle of supporters now.

Look for opportunities of social interaction that do not involve food. Get a group of friends together for a walk around a lake or at a local park. Get out your bicycle and ride to a friend's house to help her plant her garden. Grab your camera and head out with a friend who is a photography buff. You'll quickly find that food and drink can be just things that are "there" when you gather socially. What's really important are the personal interactions, the shared experiences, and the stories. Find your core group of supporters, and enlist them to help you seek out those experiences.

# Motivational Tools

Even if you're successful in cultivating a positive attitude, and you have a good group of core supporters, as you begin implementing new healthy lifestyle changes, you will encounter some pretty big obstacles along the way, and your motivation is likely to dip at times. When that happens, acknowledge that it's normal, adopt the best attitude you can, and then look for ways to bolster that attitude. Here are a few exercises you can do as needed, to help get your motivation back up and keep you going strong.

### Keep a Daily "Ideal Self" Journal

This is an advanced visualization exercise that draws on both your experiences in the present and your imagined picture of the future. Whenever you feel as though you're losing the connection to your visualized ideal self, do this journaling exercise for a week or so. Each night before you go to bed, reflect on the events of the day. Move chronologically through the day, but instead of remembering things as they happened, imagine how the day would have gone for your ideal self. How would the events of the day have been different if you were at your ideal weight now? What would life be like for the fit, thin, and healthy you? What clothes would you have worn? What activities might you have participated in that you chose not to today? Would some of the activities you did today have been easier or more enjoyable for you? How would people have talked to you and looked at you? Jot down some notes in your journal about those differences. Imagine that version of you, going through your life right now, and then get excited about it, knowing that the only thing standing between you and that imagined self is time!

### Seek Out Motivational Media

There are tons of movies, TV shows, documentaries, magazine articles, websites, and blogs that are filled with motivational content. If you're struggling with lack of motivation in a particular area, seek out sources that specifically address that subject. If you've been walking and are thinking that you'd like to try jogging if you could just get motivated enough, subscribe to a running magazine or check out a running group's website. If your diet has been regressing back to a less healthy one, stream a documentary or TED Talk series about eating fresh, healthy whole foods. If you're really having a hard time cutting back on processed sugar, seek out a blog or a social network group that addresses that issue. Believe me, if you can imagine it, it already exists somewhere. Someone else has already taken the time and done the work—you can just sit back and enjoy the motivational fruits of their labor.

## Use a Lifeline

When the going gets really tough, it's time to look to your social support network and call up somebody you can count on. Oftentimes a lack of motivation might only be due to the feeling that you're in this alone. Calling or e-mailing a friend, family member, fellow weight-loser, or your trainer and having a quick chat is probably just the thing you need to get over the bump. Hearing some encouraging words from someone important to you is a powerful thing. If your personal support network is a little thin (or if it's 2:00 a.m. and your friends are not marsupials), there are some wonderful online diet and fitness communities that have instant chat forums. You may not even need to individually connect with someone—sometimes just reading about the similar experiences of others is all it takes to get that feeling of support or the advice you were looking for.

## Ask Yourself If You Are Happy

Happiness might seem like something that will "come to you" once you've achieved your weight-loss goal, but nothing could be further from the truth. The reality is that if you are unhappy now, you're likely to struggle mightily in the pursuit of any goal you set.

Our physical health is inseparable from our mental and emotional well-being. Remember that soul-searching journal exercise in Exercise 14—Examine Deeper Root Causes? How are you coming along with addressing those issues? If you kind of glossed over that exercise, telling yourself you'd get to it later, then right about now you might be finding yourself struggling with this whole endeavor. If you are generally unhappy; if your close relationships are troubled; if you hate your job; if you've made no room in your life for play or joy or pleasure, then it won't be long until you ask yourself, "What's the point of this whole weight-loss thing anyway?" When bigger, foundational life issues are left unresolved, the condition of the physical body becomes a secondary concern, and it suffers as a result.

If you skipped Exercise 14 the first time, or if you only halfheartedly made the effort to explore your deeper issues, I encourage you to ask yourself right now, "Am I happy?" And if the answer is anything other than a resounding, unqualified "Yes!" then go back and do the exercise over again.

*Recast Yourself in a Better Role*

Who you are right now is in large part the result of how you've been viewing yourself. What label have you given yourself? Are you the funny person, there to make everyone else laugh? Are you the dependable person, putting everyone else's needs ahead of your own? Are you the super-busy, stressed-out person, just trying to hold it all together? I have news for you—you don't have to be any of these. Make the decision right now to stop being that person and start being a different one. You are the writer, producer, and director of your life's script, and you can cast yourself in any role you choose.

Society, the media, your parents, your spouse, your children, your boss—you get a lot of cues from these sources about what you "should" be doing. These can be very strong influencers, and years or decades of trying to meet their expectations has strongly reinforced the role you've been playing. By now, you may have come to view this role as your "identity," but it's not your identity, unless you continue to make it so. As an adult human being, you possess the free will that enables you to be and do whatever you want. If the role you've been playing has done you more harm than good, if it has contributed to your weight gain, your unhappiness, your poor health, your insomnia, your anxiety, your depression, then it's time to recast yourself in a better role.

Much of the work you've done in the visualization exercises has been a step in that direction, but now I want you to really think of your life as a play or a movie, with all of the important people in your life being the supporting actors in that story. What role would you give yourself if you could decide? What turn would your story take if you could write yourself the perfect script? I want you to think of it in this way because for a little while, in order to start changing, you may need to feel as though you're acting. It might be easier for you to do certain things "in character" than they would be for you to do "in real life."

Become the character that you want to be. Take on those personality traits. Be more assertive, be calm, be organized, learn to say no. And always, always, see your character in the body you want to have.

## Get More Sleep!

Ah, now here's one you likely think you don't have any control over. After all, who among us doesn't want an extra hour or two of sleep? The truth is, you almost certainly have much more time than you think you do during the day to get things done so that you can grab that extra sleep time. To see what I'm talking about, I want you to keep a time log for a few days, tracking your activities in 30-minute increments from the time you wake up to the time you fall asleep. I encourage you to use a program on your computer at home and at work that will tell you exactly how long you've spent on different task categories. These programs track your activity and break it down into "productive" and "unproductive" time based on parameters you set. I use the free version of a program called Rescue Time, but there are many others you can use. I promise, if you haven't done this before, the results will surprise you! You'll find hours of wasted time, and if you learn to structure your day better, you can use that time to get more sleep.

What does sleep have to do with weight loss anyway? A lot, actually. A research review conducted by the *Journal of the Academy of Nutrition and Dietetics* found that partial sleep deprivation negatively impacts the hormones that regulate appetite and energy balance.[2] And I'm not talking about extreme sleeplessness. The study defined partial sleep deprivation as fewer than six hours per night.[3] Seven hours is what most experts recommend as a minimum nightly goal, but many individuals may need more. This is an easy win-win. You like to sleep, and doing it more can help you lose weight! The hard part will be changing your daily habits so that you can get to bed earlier and sleep better throughout the night. Some of the things that can make you sleep poorly include watching TV or being on a computer (even reading an e-reader) within an hour of bedtime; eating within an hour or two of bedtime; drinking too much caffeine or having it too late in the day; and drinking alcohol. Learn more about how you can get a good night's sleep at http://www.helpguide.org/life/sleep_tips.htm.

## Turn Distress into De-Stress

The hormonal response to chronic stress is a complex one, and unfortunately one that works mightily against your weight-loss efforts. Repeated exposure to even mildly stressful situations pits your adrenal system against you. Your body enters a three-phase cycle that repeats itself on an endless loop until you do something to break it. First, your adrenal system falls into a chronic stress-response state, which prompts the release of certain hormonal substances (called glucocorticoids) that both increase your appetite for high-sugar, high-fat comfort foods, and simultaneously signal the body to increase its abdominal fat stores.[4] So there are really two components going on here—the one being purely hormonal and biological, and the other being behavioral ("stress eating"). The trouble is, even if you can out-will the impulse to eat poorly, you can't think away the hormonal tendencies to increase fat stores. The solution, then, is that you *must* find a way to relieve your chronic stress.

A good place to start is by simply paying attention to your body. Are your shoulders hunched around your ears? Do you clench your jaw all day long? Do you frequently feel a pang in your stomach when you think about certain people or situations? What are your nervous habits? I recommend keeping a tally sheet in your notebook and counting the number of times you catch yourself doing one of these things (or whatever your unique physical stress responses are). Then ask yourself what triggered the response. What were you thinking about or doing, who were you talking to? After a few days, you may see a pattern emerge, where one or a small handful of triggers are creating most of your stress. From this knowledge, you can take some positive action steps.

Start thinking about ways to eliminate those big stressors in your life. If it's work related (as it often is), then ask yourself some big and tough questions about whether this is what you want to be doing. If you feel that you can't afford not to, ask yourself whether your job is really worth risking your health for. Remember that you have a decision here—you *can* choose to find another job in the same industry or seek out another line of work entirely. I don't recommend quitting on the spot (unless your financial situation allows for it), as that's likely to create a whole host of other stressors, but start coming up with a plan for how you can transition from doing something you dislike to doing something that feels like more of a calling. Even just having this "escape plan" in place can change the way you feel about your job, relieving a lot of stress before you take any action at all.

The people in our lives can often be a big source of stress too, even those whom we love very much. Think about what it is that stresses you out. Is it something that person does? Is it something they expect you to do? Realize that you can never force change on someone else, but also realize that if you simply communicated about this with that person, the situation might be easily resolved. Many people are completely oblivious to the fact that they are doing something or not doing something, and you may only have to point it out in order for them to change. Of course, you'll need to use sound communication techniques and not be accusatory or defensive. Think carefully about what you'll say to your loved one and then broach the subject on neutral territory, when you're both calm, and not right after the person has done the thing you dislike.

Some stressors can't be eliminated, so they have to be coped with. There are a multitude of ways to do this, and, not surprisingly, physical activity ranks high on the list. But you don't have to do a hard-core workout every time you feel tense. Studies have shown that 30 minutes of moderate-intensity cardiovascular exercise two or three times per week can help fight stress, anxiety, and depression.[5]

Apart from physical activity, you can use breathing techniques, meditation, calming music or sounds, aromatherapy, and other relaxation techniques to combat stress. Learn more about what you can do at http://www.helpguide.org/mental/stress_management_relief_coping.htm.

## Chapter Thirteen

# MAKING IT PERMANENT

Depending on how long it's taken you to read this book up to this point and how diligent you've been in completing the exercises, you may be well on your way to achieving your weight-loss goals, or you may just be getting started. I encourage you to revisit this final chapter of the book at some point in the future, when you feel you've done the hard work and you're close to reaching your weight-loss goal.

The good news is that the hard part can be over, but only if you *take active steps* to ensure that it is. The weight you've lost can stay gone for good, but unlike a work project or a school paper, you will never really be "finished" with this process. You're better informed now about all of the influences and potential pitfalls that are out there. It would be a shame to let them sneak back into your life now, after you've worked so hard to get to this point. This chapter is intended to help you keep the weight off, placing you proudly among the ranks of the successful 20 percent.

## Look Back to the Beginning

If you began this process hoping that one day you'd reach your ideal weight and then "be done," your odds of staying at the top of the class are not very good. Remember what life was like back then—no exercise; eating bad food, too much food, stuff that was hardly food at all? All along I've been telling you that this is about lifestyle change; that you would need to come out of the process a different person than the one you were when you went in if the change was going to be permanent. Right now I'd like you to pause for a moment and look at just how far you've come and how different your life is. If you want to hold on to that, if you want to keep living life in the new role you've cast, then consistency and persistence will need to become two of your most prominent personality traits.

When thinking about weight loss, you would be better served by comparing yourself to a recovering addict than to a mountain climber setting out to summit a high peak. The climber must plan and work hard and overcome obstacles, but he eventually reaches the summit and his journey ends. The addict, on the other hand, wakes up every day facing the same challenges as the day before. Maybe you've reached your ultimate goal or you've made very good progress toward it already. If that's the case, then great congratulations are in order! But if, after congratulating yourself, you sit back now and "take it easy," you'll be surprised at how quickly your old bad habits can sneak back into your life. Looking back at where you were before should make you proud of where you are now, but it should also put you on alert. That person is someone you used to be. Your job now is to figure out how to never go back to being that person again.

## I Made It! Now What?

To get to where you are today, you've worked very hard, and you've probably had some favorable conditions working for you as well. You've learned a whole new set of skills and developed healthy habits. Those habits will not only make it likely that you'll live longer but that the quality of those extra years will be far better than they otherwise would have been. Going forward, the challenge will be to keep feeding your motivation while learning to practice extreme vigilance. How vigilant you must be and what methods you use will depend on your physical makeup, your personality, and which road you took to arrive at this wonderful place.

For example, say that you've always hated exercise, but you did it during the weight-loss phase of your program because you knew how important it was. Now that you've lost the weight, you're wondering what your options might be. You're willing to keep up some physical activity a few days per week for health benefits, but you're hoping you can scale back a bit now that you've reached the maintenance phase of your program. You *are* willing, however, to keep up the healthy eating habits you've formed over the past months, checking in regularly by tracking calories carefully in your food log. This strategy can work.

Suppose instead that you've found you don't mind working out pretty hard five or six days a week—in fact, there are one or two activities you really love. But you can't live any longer without donuts or pizza or the occasional rack of ribs. You're willing to work out like a maniac so that you don't have to eat as well as you have been during your weight-loss phase. This can also work, but it is much more dangerous than the first option, because you can consume calories more quickly than you can burn them.

In either case, you can only let up in one area, not both, and you must be very aware of the caloric impact that any changes in diet or activity will have.

Extreme vigilance involves very close oversight on your part. You'll need to weigh in several times a week—I suggest daily—and at the first sign of weight gain, you'll need to assess what's causing that, probably by food logging for a week or two. In short, being vigilant means that you are *actively measuring* how well you're maintaining your new, healthy lifestyle.

In this maintenance stage, while it is possible to relax a bit where diet and exercise are concerned, it's very important to distinguish between the *small* increases in calorie consumption you may allow yourself now and the kind of eating and drinking you were doing before you started the program. There is simply no going back there, ever. You were *gaining* weight then, remember? Losing weight lowers your metabolism—it's just a fact. When you weigh less, your body simply doesn't need as much energy to drag itself around. What's more, this reduced rate of energy expenditure appears to be permanent.[1]

This means you'll have to decide what stays and what goes. You can give up an hour or so of exercise per week as long as you're willing to eat really well (and you may have to track your calories), or you can eat more of what you really want, but only if you're willing to continue a rigorous exercise regimen, or even step it up a notch. I personally do a little of both. I eat better than the general population, but I don't deny myself small and occasional samplings of foods that are nothing but bad for me. Also, even though I do eat quite healthfully most of the time, I eat frequently and in fairly big portions. I make up for that by exercising for at least 30 minutes (usually an hour) almost *every* day. This is the part where you get to decide what the best combination is for you. But don't think that just making the decision means you will automatically stick to it. You've got to be vigilant!

## Halfway There and Stuck!

If you've lost a significant amount of weight, but still have a ways to go, the situation is different. What I alluded to but didn't come right out and say in chapter 9 is that for most people, this is a process that happens in stages, with many stops and starts. What is important is that you regard the stops as short pauses rather than as long-term regressions or failures. Hold on to the progress you've made and keep the essential elements of your new healthy habits in play. Remember that your main focus during a plateau is to *give nothing back*! You've earned those lost pounds, so don't let frustration and impatience cause you to give up and regress to past behavior patterns. Acknowledge that things won't be as great as they were in the early days of high motivation and fast progress, but you *will* continue to make progress, and that is ultimately how you will reach your goals.

Weight loss will continue to happen in chunks here and there, and I hate to tell you, but there may even be some small weight gains spattered along the way. Expect those moments and confront them rationally, rather than emotionally. Acknowledge your disappointment and frustration, and then move on, finding new ways around the barriers and toward your goals.

In chapter 9, I talked about a couple of ways to deal with short-term plateaus, but you should know that some pauses can be very long—like, years long! You might even find yourself saying, "Well, I've lost a lot of weight, I feel a lot better, and I look pretty good." It is just fine, and possibly even advisable, to knowingly take a month-long break from weight loss. Just be sure that you *give nothing back*, and maintain your weight by keeping up your healthy habits. Then one day when you get a second wind or start a new activity or experience a shift in your metabolism, you'll continue on toward your goal again.

Ten years ago, when I was about 10 to 15 pounds heavier than my current (and ideal) weight, I thought, *Well, I've lost 30 pounds and I look and feel really good. I've still got some problem areas, but all in all, I'm pretty happy with things the way they are.* At that point in time, I thought I ate pretty healthfully and couldn't imagine cooking as much as I do now. But it turned out that cooking became an activity I truly loved. At its best, I find cooking to be a zen-like experience, combining creative expression and present-moment relaxation. At its worst, it's a labor that has both immediate and long-term payoffs and is still worth the time and effort.

On the exercise front, I never imagined that I would take up running as a serious hobby, much less ever run a marathon, but when the idea of it first popped into my head, rather than shooting it down as an absurdity, I entertained it, mulled it over for a few days, and then committed wholly to it in one big, head-first dive. It turned out that the combination of my healthy cooking hobby along with my marathon training were what ultimately shed those last 10 pounds for me.

Does this mean that you'll have to run a marathon and spend hours cooking every week in order to reach your ideal weight? Nope, but you probably will have to find your own combination of "next-level habits" to make it happen.

## Next-Level Habits

"Next-level habits" are those extra-mile steps you might have to take in order to overcome a big plateau and ultimately reach your final weight-loss goal. They can also be thought of as secret weapons you can use to get your motivation back on track if you've slipped a little and what worked before is no longer working. They might also apply if your reasons for wanting to lose weight have shifted from physical and mental health-related ones to those based a little more on vanity. Hey, there's nothing wrong with a little vanity—it can be a very strong positive motivator, and as long as it's not taken too far, I suggest you use it to your advantage!

Perhaps you don't care much about taking off those last 10 or 15 pounds. You look and feel great, you're at a much lower risk for chronic disease, and so you've decided to call it done and shift into permanent maintenance mode. If this is the case, then you have succeeded and you should feel proud! If, on the other hand, you have caught a glimpse of what could be and you want to go for it, then dig in and be ready to fight—those last 10 pounds can be the most stubborn!

The truth is, you probably won't reach your ultimate goal by doing what has gotten you to this point. Rather, you'll need to step up your effort and engagement, but this is actually where things can get really fun! Here are just a few next-level habits you can strive for, any one of which might be enough to take you down the home stretch and get you all the way to your goal.

### Become an Athlete

Taking up a sport can be a fast-track way to burn those last few pounds of fat. The good news is that even if you don't feel very confident in your fitness or ability, there is almost certainly a club or league or class designed for people at exactly your level.

There is likely to be a very wide range of options for just about any sport you choose, and once you figure out what you want to do, you'll be surprised by the big welcome you'll get from others with similar interests. There are basketball and volleyball leagues, running and cycling clubs, racquetball and handball leagues, hiking and walking groups, and a host of other sports and activities out there with groups already established that you will fit right into.

Aside from the calories you'll burn, taking up a sport can offer so many other amazing benefits. You will feel a strong sense of belonging; you'll begin to identify yourself as an athlete; you will expand your circle of friends; there will be an added layer of accountability for you. So if you've been kicking around the idea of starting or taking back up a particular sport, take the next step and start looking for groups or leagues in your area. Active meet-up groups, your local YMCA, or the independent running store or bike shop in your town are all great places to start looking.

### Be a Mentor

Maybe you've already taken up running or cycling or you participate in a particular sport or activity. Chances are, there is an organization nearby looking for adults to mentor kids, and what better way to spend time with a young person than by doing something active? There are even nonprofit groups out there whose primary mission is to introduce healthy physical activity into kids' lives in the form of organized after-school or summer activities.

By taking on a role of responsibility, you up the ante—there's no slacking now, because someone else is looking at you to see what they should be doing. Sharing your story with young people, or even other adults who are at square one and looking for guidance and encouragement, is not only extra motivation for you, it's invaluable to them.

### Take a Course or Attend a Clinic

There are a ton of low-cost and free educational opportunities popping up all over the place, but none more comprehensive than the MOOCs: Massive Open Online Courses, which are offered by a number of prestigious universities via the Internet. Many of these schools offer six-, eight-, or twelve-week courses covering a number of topics related to weight loss, be it nutrition, exercise physiology, or athletic performance. You can gain a lot of great knowledge and plenty of motivation for free, and on your own schedule.

If you can't commit to a multi-week course, there are probably a good handful of two- or three-hour classes covering similar topics offered through your local Community Education department. Not only that, but cooking supply stores, co-operative markets, and even traditional grocery stores are starting to offer classes that are free or very low-cost. Many of these classes will help you learn basic cooking skills, if you don't already have them, and many are specifically geared toward using healthier cooking methods and ingredients.

If you'd like to boost your knowledge and motivation in the exercise arena, Community Ed or your local fitness center are good places to learn about things like yoga, weight lifting, and more. If you're interested in a particular sport, look for area gyms that are offering skills clinics where seasoned professionals will teach you how you can up your game. If you're into cycling, take a bicycle repair class at the local bike shop. Whatever your area of interest, there's nothing more motivating than spending a few hours with a group of people who are as into it as you are. This is also a great place to look for others at your ability level and join or form a meet-up group.

### Take a Challenge (or Make Your Own)

In a way, a challenge is a lot like setting a goal, but it's a very limited, very specific goal. You'll want to pick something you're having a hard time with and set clear rules for yourself, but then make a deadline—an end to the challenge, after which you don't need to follow it as strictly, or at all. This might sound like it runs counter to the whole "lifestyle change" thing, but short-term challenges can actually serve as great first steps toward making tough changes that just seem impossible when viewed through the lens of "for the rest of my life."

You've likely seen a few challenges floating around on social media. These are things like "100 Push-ups" or "30 Days of Squats." Be cautious here; many of these are not a very good idea for even quite fit individuals, so if you're still not in great shape, it's probably best to skip them altogether. Often, though, you can modify the parameters of a popular challenge so that you are still able to participate with your friends on social media, and this can be very motivational. For example, instead of doing one hundred push-ups every day, maybe you start with twenty and work your way up to fifty.

It's probably better, though, to make your own specific challenge that targets one of your trouble spots. For example, let's say you've been having a really hard time getting in five workouts each week. A good challenge that might move you toward overcoming this obstacle is to say, "I am going to exercise *every day* for the next *two weeks*." Because the challenge is bound by a short timeline, you're much more likely to find a way to get those fourteen workouts in. And when you get to the end of the challenge, you'll have to admit that if you could exercise *every day* for two weeks, then it shouldn't be so hard for you to get in five workouts a week on a more long-term basis. You should see a big improvement on your exercise calendar in the weeks that follow, and if you find yourself slipping again a few months down the line, then you can do this challenge again or come up with another one.

I have done some pretty crazy challenges myself (and I always invite my clients and blog subscribers to join me). One of my challenges was to log one million steps on my pedometer in one hundred days (ten thousand steps a day, every day for one hundred days straight). I hit the million-step mark at 9:00 a.m. on the morning my challenge was ending. Another year I did a "365 Days of Activity" challenge: I did something active for at least 20 minutes *every single day for one whole year.* It was hard! There were days when I was sick, tired, injured, or just plain unmotivated.

But I always found *something* I could do, whether it was a short restorative yoga session, a slow walk with my dogs, or an easy resistance band workout.

As I said, those are some extreme examples of exercise-related challenges, but they are just two examples of the kinds of things you can come up with. Use your own imagination and find ways to tackle stubborn problems you are up against. (Both of my challenges were intended to make me be more consistent with my own exercise routine, and they worked!)

In chapter 11, I mentioned the Rainbow Challenge and Whole Grains Challenge. But you can carry a dietary challenge much further than that. Imagine a *perfect* day of eating, based on the type of diet you've chosen to follow. Walk yourself through that day and think about what you'd have for breakfast, lunch, dinner, and the little meals in between. What would you drink? How would you get in your five to nine servings of fruits and vegetables? What kinds of foods, prepared in what way, would be the most nourishing for your body? Now do it.

Write out a one-day meal plan answering the questions above. Search for and select the most delicious, nutritious recipes you can find, then take stock of what you have on hand and make a shopping list for the rest of it. Go to the store and carefully select only the best ingredients. Then pick a day in the next week when you can put your plan into action. For one entire day, eat *perfectly*. Keep notes in your journal about how you felt that day. What was the food like? Did you enjoy preparing it? What might you change the next time you do this? Is this something you could stretch out into two or three days?

By going to extremes, we challenge ourselves to move beyond our comfort zones. Our old "best efforts" can suddenly have lots of room for improvement when we push ourselves far beyond them, even if only for one day. While a one-day experiment or challenge will not result in lasting behavior change, it can serve as a powerful prod to motivate us to do a little more on a daily basis, and that *can* have permanent effects.

Regardless of what kind of challenge you do or for how long, one trick you can use to get an even bigger benefit from it is to go public. Tell your friends and family about it, and even ask them to join you. Participating in an activity as part of a group is always more motivational than doing it by yourself, and having the added layer of accountability can only up your chances for a successful outcome.

# IN PARTING

If you've been working hard and doing the exercises outlined in the first part of the book, then I'm sure you've made great progress by now. You are somewhere along the path of transforming yourself from who you once were into that ideal self you know you can be. Congratulations!

The physical body is certainly not the whole person—there is much more to you than what meets the world's eye—but it is the part that *you show to the world*, your physical representation of who you are. Not only that, but it's the part that carries you through this wonderful thing called life. Don't let that part of you be a victim of circumstance any longer. Don't let the experience of life be anything less than remarkable. Know that you've taken control and you're changing things on a cellular level. By changing your pattern of behaviors, you really can reboot your body, rewriting its code by getting in "above genetics" to literally alter your physical makeup.

Every single person reading these words has the capacity to make those changes. The only thing that can ever stop you is you. So don't be your own road block. Be persistent, do the work, stay motivated, and applaud yourself as you see the person you were melt away and transform into the person you really want to show to the rest of the world.

My greatest hope is that this book has been a useful tool in your weight-loss efforts. If it has, I'd love to hear from you. You can connect with me online at www.wellcuratedlife.com/contact. I look forward to hearing about how you are rebooting your body!

# NOTES

## Introduction

1. Cheng, Z. & Almeida, F. A. Mitochondrial alteration in type 2 diabetes and obesity: An epigenetic link. *Cell Cycle* 2014, 13, 890–897. Retrieved from https://www.landesbioscience.com/journals/cc /2013CC5448R.pdf.

2. Kelly, M. Weapons of fat mass destruction. Retrieved from https://www.acefitness.org/continuing education/courses/webexcourse.aspx?courseID=WEB-WFMD-10&WebExamID=476149&CustN mbr=N300088&AID=4a527yxx.

3. Duin, J. (November 10, 2011). Snake handling is still considered a sign of faith. *Washington Post Magazine*. Retrieved from http://www.washingtonpost.com/lifestyle/magazine/in-wva-snake -handling-is-still-considered-a-sign-of-faith/2011/10/18/gIQAmiqL9M_story.html.

4. Goleman, D. (June 28, 1988). Probing the enigma of multiple personality. The *New York Times* Archives. Retrieved from http://www.nytimes.com/1988/06/28/science/probing-the-enigma-of -multiple-personality.html?pagewanted=all&src=pm.

5. McRae, C. et al. (2004). Effects of perceived treatment on quality of life and medical outcomes in a double-blind placebo surgery trial. *JAMA Psychiatry*, 61(6), 627. Retrieved from http://archpsyc .jamanetwork.com/article.aspx?articleid=481982.

6. Brody, H. & Miller, F. G. (2011). Lessons from recent research about the placebo effect—from art to science. *Journal of the American Medical Association*, 306(23), 2612–2613. Retrieved from http:// jama.jamanetwork.com/article.aspx?articleid=1104739.

7. See Jog, M. S. et al. (1999). Building neural representations of habits. Science, 286, 1745. doi: 10.1126 /science.286.5445.1745. Retrieved from http://web.mit.edu/bcs/graybiel-lab/publications/Science_ Jog.pdf; Dezfouli, A. & Balleine, B. W. (2012). Habits, action sequences and reinforcement learning. The *European Journal of Neuroscience*, 35(7), 1036–1051. Retrieved from http://www.ncbi.nlm.nih .gov/pmc/articles/PMC3325518/ ; Rönn, T. et al. (June 27, 2013). A six months exercise intervention influences the genome-wide DNA methylation pattern in human adipose tissue. *PLOS Genetics*. doi: 10.1371/journal.pgen.1003572; Howe, S. (October 14, 2013). Epigenetics: How our lifestyle can impact our genes. iRunFar.com. Retrieved from http://www.irunfar.com/2013/10/epigenetics-how -our-lifestyle-can-impact-our-genes.html. Ornish, D. (December 3, 2008). Changing Lifestyle Changes Gene Expression. Edge.org. Retrieved from http://edge.org/conversation/changing -lifestyle-changes-gene-expression

## Prologue

1. Bryant, C. X. et al. (2013). *ACE Health Coach Manual*. (San Diego, CA: American Council on Exercise), 202.

2. Ibid.

3. Centers for Disease Control and Prevention. A Snapshot: Diabetes in the United States. Retrieved from http://www.cdc.gov/diabetes/pubs/statsreport14/diabetes-infographic.pdf.

4. Hurt, R. T. et al. (2010). The obesity epidemic: Challenges, health initiatives, and implications for gastroenterologists. *Gastroenterology & Hepatology*, 6(12), 780–792. Retrieved from http://www.ncbi.nlm.nih.gov/pmc/articles/PMC3033553/.

5. Olansky, S. J. et al. (2005). A potential decline in life expectancy in the United States in the 21st century. *New England Journal of Medicine*, 352, 1138-114. doi: 10.1056/NEJMsr043743. Retrieved from http://www.nejm.org/doi/full/10.1056/NEJMsr043743.

6. Cawley, J. & Maclean, J. C. (September 2010). Unfit for service: The implications of rising obesity for U.S. military recruitment. National Bureau of Economic Research Working Paper, No. 16408. Retrieved from http://www.nber.org/papers/w16408.

7. Barlas, F. M. et al. (February 2013). Overview of key measures of healthy lifestyle and disease prevention. 2011 Department of Defense Health Related Behaviors Survey of Active Duty Military Personnel. 32-45. Fairfax, VA: ICF International. Retrieved from https://www.documentcloud.org/documents/694942-2011-final-department-of-defense-survey-of.html

8. Urbana High School Agricultural Basic Mechanics. (2007). The Internal Combustion Engine and Its Importance to Agriculture. Retrieved from http://uhsagbm.wikispaces.com/file/view/020107.pdf.

9. Carlson, M. (June 12, 2008). Earl Butz. The Guardian online. Retrieved from http://www.theguardian.com/world/2008/feb/04/usa.obituaries.

10. Ibid.; Agriculture in the Classroom. Growing a Nation: The Story of American Agriculture. Retrieved from http://www.agclassroom.org/gan/timeline/1970.htm.

11. Reisner, R. & Thompson, D. (January 10, 2008). The diet industry: A big fat lie. Bloomberg Businessweek online. Retrieved from http://www.businessweek.com/debateroom/archives/2008/01/the_diet_indust.html.

12. Muniz, K. (March 24, 2014). 20 ways Americans are blowing their money. The Motley Fool. Retrieved from http://www.usatoday.com/story/money/personalfinance/2014/03/24/20-ways-we-blow-our-money/6826633/.

13. Nestle 2013 Annual Report, 55. (2014). Nestle S. A., Cham & Vevey (Switzerland). Retrieved from http://www.nestle.com/asset-library/documents/library/documents/annual_reports/2013-annual-report-en.pdf.

14. Nestle 2013 Annual Report, 55, 64. (2014). Nestle S. A., Cham and Vevey (Switzerland). Retrieved from http://www.nestle.com/asset-library/documents/library/documents/annual_reports/2013-annual-report-en.pd.

15. American Diabetes Association online. (2013). The Cost of Diabetes. Retrieved from http://www.diabetes.org/advocacy/news-events/cost-of-diabetes.html.

16. Speers, S. et al. (April 2011). Child and adolescent exposure to food and beverage brand appearances during prime-time television programming. *American Journal of Preventive Medicine*, 41(3), 291–296. Retrieved from http://www.ajpmonline.org/cms/attachment/2000865584/2002810542/mmc1.pdf.

17. Nixon, R. (February 20, 2012). New guidelines planned on school vending machines. *The New York Times* online. Retrieved from http://www.nytimes.com/2012/02/21/us/politics/new-rules -planned-on-school-vending-machines.html?_r=0.

18. World Health Organization online. (August 2014). Obesity and overweight. Fact Sheet No. 311. Retrieved from http://www.who.int/mediacentre/factsheets/fs311/en/.

19. Farooqi, I. S. & O'Rahilly, S. (2007), Genetic factors in human obesity. *Obesity Reviews*, 8, 37–40. doi: 10.1111/j.1467-789X.2007.00315.x. Retrieved from http://onlinelibrary.wiley.com/doi/10.1111/j .1467-789X.2007.00315.x/full.

20. Cheng, Z. & Almeida, F. A. Mitochondrial alteration in type 2 diabetes and obesity: An epigenetic link. *Cell Cycle*, 2014; 13, 890–897. Retrieved from https://www.landesbioscience.com/journals/cc/2013 CC5448R.pdf; Ornish, D. et al. (June 17, 208). Changes in prostate gene expression in men undergoing an intensive nutrition and lifestyle intervention. *Proceedings of the National Academy of Sciences United States of America.*, 105(24), 8369–8374. Retrieved from http://www.pnas.org/content/105/24/8369.full; Ornish, D. (December 3, 2008). Changing lifestyle changes gene expression. Edge.org. Retrieved from http://edge.org/conversation/changing-lifestyle-changes-gene-expression.

21. Mattmiller, B. (December 10, 2007). Genome study places modern humans in the evolutionary fast lane. *University of Wisconsin-Madison News*. Retrieved from http://www.news.wisc.edu/14548.

22. Wing, R. & Phelan, S. (2005). Long-term weight loss maintenance. *American Journal of Clinical Nutrition* 82, 222S–225S. Retrieved from http://ajcn.nutrition.org/content/82/1/222S.long.

## Part 1: Your Structural Roadmap to Permanent Weight Loss

1. Ornish, D. et al. (June 17, 2008). Changes in prostate gene expression in men undergoing an intensive nutrition and lifestyle intervention. *Proceedings of the National Academy of Sciences United States of America*, 105(24), 8369–8374. Retrieved from https://www.landesbioscience.com /journals/cc/2013CC5448R.pdf; Ornish, D. et al. (Sep 16, 2008). Increased telomerase activity and comprehensive lifestyle changes: A pilot study. *Lancet Oncology*, 9, 1048–57. doi:10.1016/S1470 -2045(08)70234-1. Retrieved from http://www.ornishspectrum.com/wp-content/uploads /increased-telomerase-activity-and-comprehensive-lifestyle-changes.pdf.

2. Ornish, D. (December 3, 2008). Changing lifestyle changes gene expression. Edge.org. Retrieved from http://edge.org/conversation/changing-lifestyle-changes-gene-expression.

3. Rönn, T. et al. (June 27, 2013). A six months exercise intervention influences the genome-wide DNA methylation pattern in human adipose tissue. *PLOS Genetics*. doi: 10.1371/journal.pgen.1003572. Retrieved from http://www.plosgenetics.org/article/info%3Adoi%2F10.1371%2Fjournal.pgen .1003572; Howe, S. (October 14, 2013). Epigenetics: How our lifestyle can impact our genes. iRunFar.com. Retrieved from http://www.irunfar.com/2013/10/epigenetics-how-our-lifestyle-can -impact-our-genes.html.

4. Jog, M. S. et al. (1999). Building neural representations of habits. *Science*, 286: 1745. doi: 10.1126 /science.286.5445.1745. Retrieved from http://web.mit.edu/bcs/graybiel-lab/publications/Science _Jog.pdf; Dezfouli, A and Balleine, B. W. (2012). Habits, action sequences and reinforcement learning. *European Journal of Neuroscience*, 35(7), 1036–1051. Retrieved from http://www.ncbi.nlm.nih.gov/pmc /articles/PMC3325518/.

# Chapter 1

1. Woods, C. et al. (2002). Physical activity intervention: A transtheoretical model-based intervention designed to help sedentary young adults become active. *Health Education Research*, 17 (4), 451–460. doi: 10.1093/her/17.4.451. Retrieved from http://her.oxfordjournals.org/content/17/4/451.full.

2. Bryant, C. X. et al. (2013), *ACE Health Coach Manual.* (San Diego, CA: American Council on Exercise), 59, 61.

3. Blackwell, S. E. et al. (2013). Optimism and mental imagery: A possible cognitive marker to promote well-being? *Psychiatry Research*, 206(1), 56–61. Retrieved from http://www.ncbi.nlm.nih.gov/pmc /articles/PMC3605581/; Peters, M. L. et al. (2010). Manipulating optimism: Can imagining a best possible self be used to increase positive future expectancies? *Journal of Positive Psychology*, 5(3), 204–211. doi: 10.1080/17439761003790963. Retrieved from http://www.tandfonline.com/doi/ full/10.1080/17439761003790963#.VFqJ64ceXzI.

4. Bryant, C. X. et al. (2013). *ACE Health Coach Manual.* (San Diego, CA: American Council on Exercise), 69.

5. Christakis, N. & Fowler, J. (July 26, 2007). The spread of obesity in a large social network over 32 years. *New England Journal of Medicine*, 357, 370–379. doi: 10.1056/NEJMsa066082. Retrieved from http://www.nejm.org/doi/full/10.1056/NEJMsa066082.

6. Hruschka, D. et al. (December 2011). Shared norms and their explanation for the social clustering of obesity. *American Journal of Public Health*, 101, S295–S300. doi: 10.2105/AJPH.2010.300053. Retrieved from http://ajph.aphapublications.org/doi/full/10.2105/AJPH.2010.300053.

# Chapter 2

1. Breton, E. et al. (September 13, 2011). Weight loss—there is an app for that! But does it adhere to evidence-informed practices? *Translational Behavioral Medicine*, 1(4): 523–529. doi: 10.1007/s13142 -011-0076-5. Retrieved from http://www.ncbi.nlm.nih.gov/pmc/articles/PMC3717669/; National Weight Control Registry online. *NWCR Facts.* Retrieved from http://www.nwcr.ws/Research /default.htm.

2. Nestle, M. (March 28, 2012). Why calories count: The problem with dietary-intake studies. *The Atlantic* online. Retrieved from http://www.theatlantic.com/health/archive/2012/03/why-calories -count-the-problem-with-dietary-intake-studies/254886/.

3. Ibid.

4. Archer, E. et al. (October 9, 2013). Validity of U.S. nutritional surveillance: National health and nutrition examination survey caloric energy intake data, 1971–2010. *PLOS One.* doi: 10.1371/journal .pone.0076632 . Retrieved from http://www.plosone.org/article/info%3Adoi%2F10.1371%2Fjournal .pone.0076632.

5. Burke, L. E. et al. (2011). Self-monitoring in weight loss: A systematic review of the literature. *Journal of the American Dietetic Association*, 111(1), 92–102. Retrieved from http://www.ncbi.nlm.nih.gov/pmc /articles/PMC3268700/.

# Chapter 3

1. Centers for Disease Control and Prevention. *Losing Weight: What Is Healthy Weight Loss?* Retrieved from http://www.cdc.gov/healthyweight/losing_weight/index.html.

2. Hall, K. et al. (April 2012). Energy balance and its components: Implications for body weight regulation. *American Journal of Clinical Nutrition*, 95(4), 989–994. doi: 10.3945/ ajcn.112.036350. Retrieved from http://ajcn.nutrition.org/content/95/4/989.short.

3. West, D. S. et al. (2011). A motivation-focused weight loss maintenance program is an effective alternative to a skill-based approach. *International Journal of Obesity*, 35, 259–269. doi: 10.1038/ijo .2010.138. Retrieved from http://www.nature.com/ijo/journal/v35/n2/abs/ijo2010138a.html.

## Chapter 4

1. Mann, T. et al. (2007). Medicare's search for effective obesity treatments: Diets are not the answer. *American Psychologist*, 62(3), 220–233. doi: 10.1037/0003-066X. Retrieved from http://motivatedandfit .com/wp-content/uploads/2010/03/Diets_dont_work.pdf.

2. National Heart, Lung and Blood Institute, online. (Updated June 2014). What Is the DASH Eating Plan? Retrieved from http://www.nhlbi.nih.gov/health/health-topics/topics/dash/

3. Ganz, M. et al. (2014). The association of body mass index with the risk of type 2 diabetes: A case–control study nested in an electronic health records system in the United States. *Diabeteology & Metabolic Syndrome*, 6, 50. doi: 10.1186/1758-5996-6-50. Retrieved from http://www.dmsjournal .com/content/6/1/50.

4. Barr, S. & Wright, J. (2010). Postprandial energy expenditure in whole-food and processed-food meals: Implications for daily energy expenditure. *Food and Nutrition Research*, 54. doi: 10.3402/fnr .v54i0.5144. Retrieved from http://www.ncbi.nlm.nih.gov/pmc/articles/PMC2897733/.

5. Tuso, P. et al. (2013). Nutritional update for physicians: Plant-based diets. *Permanente Journal*, 17(2), 61–66. Retrieved from http://www.ncbi.nlm.nih.gov/pmc/articles/PMC3662288/.

6. Trapp, C. & Levin, S. (February 2012). Preparing to prescribe plant-based diets for diabetes prevention and treatment. *Diabetes Spectrum*, 25(1), 38–44. Retrieved from http://spectrum.diabetesjournals.org /content/25/1/38.full.pdf+html.

7. Estruch, R. et al. (2013). Primary prevention of cardiovascular disease with a Mediterranean diet. *New England Journal of Medicine*, 368, 1279–1290. doi: 10.1056/NEJMoa1200303. Retrieved from http://www.nejm.org/doi/full/10.1056/NEJMoa1200303; Samieri, C. et al. (2013). The relation of midlife diet to healthy aging: A cohort study. *Annals of Internal Medicine*, 159(9), 584–591. Retrieved from http://www.ncbi.nlm.nih.gov/pmc/articles/PMC4193807/.

8. Samieri, C. et al. (2013). The relation of midlife diet to healthy aging: A cohort study. *Annals of Internal Medicine*, 159(9), 584–591. Retrieved from http://www.ncbi.nlm.nih.gov/pmc/articles /PMC4193807/; Alcalay, R. N. et al. (2012). The association between Mediterranean diet adherence and Parkinson's disease. *Movement Disorders*, 27(6), 771–774. doi: 10.1002/mds.24918. Retrieved from http://www.ncbi.nlm.nih.gov/pmc/articles/PMC3349773/; Psaltopoulou, T. et al. (2013). Mediterranean diet, stroke, cognitive impairment, and depression: A meta-analysis. *Annals of Neurology*, 74(4), 580–591. doi: 10.1002/ana.23944. Retrieved from http://www.nutrociencia.com .br/upload_files/artigos_download/ana23944.pdf;

9. Alcalay, R. N. et al. (2012). The association between Mediterranean diet adherence and Parkinson's disease. *Movement Disorders*, 27(6), 771–774. doi: 10.1002/mds.24918 http://www.ncbi.nlm.nih.gov /pmc/articles/PMC3349773/.

10. Westerterp-Plantenga, M. et al. (2012). Dietary protein: Its role in satiety, energetics, weight loss and health. *British Journal of Nutrition*, 108, S105–S112. Retrieved from http://journals.cambridge .org/download.php?file=%2FBJN%2FBJN108_S2%2FS0007114512002589a.pdf&code=af0ce 26fdd6a14d39f1f376d4cb1ef35; Wycherley, T. et al. (2010). A high-protein diet with resistance exercise training improves weight loss and body composition in overweight and obese patients with type 2 diabetes. *Diabetes Care*, 33(5), 969–976. doi: 10.2337/dc09-1974. Retrieved from http:// care.diabetesjournals.org/content/33/5/969.full; Paddon-Jones, D. et al. (2008). Protein, weight management, and satiety. *American Journal of Clinical Nutrition*, 87(5), 1558S–1561S. Retrieved from http://ajcn.nutrition.org/content/87/5/1558S.long.

11. Westerterp, K. (2004). Diet induced thermogenesis. *Nutrition & Metabolism,* 1:5. doi:10.1186/1743 -7075-1-5. Retrieved from http://www.nutritionandmetabolism.com/content/1/1/5.

12. Bryant, C. X. et al. (2013). *ACE Health Coach Manual. (*San Diego, CA: American Council on Exercise), 126.

13. Barr, S. & Wright, J. (2010). Postprandial energy expenditure in whole-food and processed-food meals: Implications for daily energy expenditure. *Food and Nutrition Research*, 54. doi: 10.3402/fnr .v54i0.5144. Retrieved from http://www.ncbi.nlm.nih.gov/pmc/articles/PMC2897733/; Whitehurst, L. (October 17, 2013). Brigham Young University study: Fight fat on cellular level? *The Salt Lake Tribune*. Retrieved from http://www.sltrib.com/sltrib/news/57010794-78/ceramide-weight-diet -cells.html.csp; Smith, M. et al. (2013). Mitochondrial fission mediates ceramide-induced metabolic disruption in skeletal muscle. *Biochemical Journal*, 456(3), 427–439. doi:10.1042 /BJ20130807. Retrieved from http://www.biochemj.org/bj/456/bj4560427.htm.

# Chapter 5

1. Schubert, M. et al. (2014). Acute exercise and hormones related to appetite regulation: A meta-analysis. *Sports Medicine*, 44(3), 387–403. Retrieved from http://www.ncbi.nlm.nih.gov/pubmed/24174308; Sim, A. Y. et al. (2013). High-intensity intermittent exercise attenuates ad-libitum energy intake. *International Journal of Obesity*. June 4, 2013. doi:10.1038/ijo.2013.102. Retrieved from http://www .ncbi.nlm.nih.gov/pubmed/23835594.

2. King, N. A. et al. (2011). Exercise, appetite and weight management: Understanding the compensatory responses in eating behavior and how they contribute to variability in exercise-induced weight loss. *British Journal of Sports Medicine*, May 19, 2011. doi:10.1136/bjsm.2010.082495. Retrieved from http:// www98.griffith.edu.au/dspace/bitstream/handle/10072/44241/75992_1.pdf?sequence=1.

3. Kerksick, C. et al. (2009). Effects of a popular exercise and weight loss program on weight loss, body composition, energy expenditure and health in obese women. *Nutrition & Metabolism*, 6, 23. doi:10.1186/1743-7075-6-23. Retrieved from http://www.nutritionandmetabolism.com/content /6/1/23; McQueen, M. A. (2009). Exercise aspects of obesity treatment. *The Ochsner Journal*, 9(3), 140–143. Retrieved from http://www.ncbi.nlm.nih.gov/pmc/articles/PMC3096271/.

4. Rönn, T. et al. (2013). A six months exercise intervention influences the genome-wide DNA methylation pattern in human adipose tissue. *PLOS Genetics*, 9(6), e1003572. doi: 10.1371/journal .pgen.1003572. Retrieved from http://www.plosgenetics.org/article/info%3Adoi%2F10.1371%2F journal.pgen.1003572.

5. Tate, D. et al. (2007). Long-term weight losses associated with prescription of higher physical activity goals. Are higher levels of physical activity protective against weight regain? *American Journal of Clinical Nutrition*, 85(4), 954–959. Retrieved from http://ajcn.nutrition.org/content /85/4/954.long; Chaput, J. P et al. (2011). Physical activity plays an important role in body weight regulation. *Journal of Obesity*. Vol. 2011 (online). dx.doi.org/10.1155/2011/360257. Retrieved from http://www.hindawi.com/journals/jobe/2011/360257/.

6. Caudwell, P. et al (2011). The influence of physical activity on appetite control: an experimental system to understand the relationship between exercise-induced energy expenditure and energy intake. *Proceedings of the Nutrition Society*, 2011(70), 171–180. doi:10.1017/S0029665110004751. Retrieved from http://journals.cambridge.org/download.php?file=%2FPNS%2FPNS70_02%2FS0 029665110004751a.pdf&code=e3fb1387a7ba96d08a9e7b504bdd5319.

7. Egan, B. & Zierath, J. R. (2012). Exercise metabolism and the molecular regulation for skeletal muscle adaptation. *Cell Metabolism*, 17(2), 162–184. doi: 10.1016/j.cmet.2012.12.012. Retrieved fromhttp://www.sciencedirect.com/science/article/pii/S1550413112005037; Department of Health & Human Services. (2008). 2008 physical activity guidelines for Americans. *At-a-Glance: A Fact Sheet for Professionals*. Retrieved from http://www.health.gov/paguidelines/pdf/fs_prof.pdf.

8. Net and gross calorie calculations computed using the metabolic calculator at http://www.exrx.net /Calculators/WalkRunMETs.html.

## Chapter 6

1. Neumark-Sztainer, D. et al. (2012). Dieting and unhealthy weight control behaviors during adolescence: Associations with 10-year changes in body mass index. *Journal of Adolescent Health*, 50(1), 80–86. Retrieved from http://www.ncbi.nlm.nih.gov/pmc/articles/PMC3245517/; Lowe, M. R. et al. (2013). Dieting and restrained eating as prospective predictors of weight gain. *Frontiers in Psychology*, 2013(4), 577–595. doi: 10.3389/fpsyg.2013.00577. Retrieved from http://www.ncbi.nlm .nih.gov/pmc/articles/PMC3759019/.

2. Anderson, E. K. et al. (2013). Weight Cycling Increases T-Cell Accumulation in Adipose Tissue and Impairs Systemic Glucose Tolerance. *Diabetes*, 62(9), 3180–3188. doi: 10.2337/db12-1076. Retrieved from http://diabetes.diabetesjournals.org/content/62/9/3180.full.

3. Cereda, E. et al. (2011). Weight cycling is associated with body weight excess and abdominal fat accumulation: A cross-sectional study. *Clinical Nutrition*, 30(6), 718–723. doi: 10.1016/j.clnu.2011 .06.009. Retrieved from http://www.sciencedirect.com/science/article/pii/S0261561411001105.

## Chapter 7

1. Saeed, A. et al. (2010). Exercise, yoga, and meditation for depressive and anxiety disorders. *American Family Physician*, 81(8), 981–986. Retrieved from http://www.aafp.org/afp/2010/0415/p981.html; Cornelissen, V. et al. (2010). Effects of aerobic training intensity on resting, exercise and post-exercise blood pressure, heart rate and heart-rate variability. *Journal of Human Hypertension*, 24, 175–182. doi: 10.1038/jhh.2009.51. Retrieved from http://www.nature.com/jhh/journal/v24/n3/full/jhh200951a.html.

2. Smith, K. S. & Graybiel, A. M. (2013). Using optogenetics to study habits. *Brain Research*, 1511: 102–114. doi: 10.1016/j.brainres.2013.01.00. Retrieved from http://www.ncbi.nlm.nih.gov/pmc /articles/PMC3654045/.

3. Centers for Disease Control and Prevention online. (Updated March 3, 2014). Physical activity. *How Much Physical Activity do Adults Need?* Retrieved from http://www.cdc.gov/physicalactivity /everyone/guidelines/adults.html.

4. The National Weight Control Registry online. *NWCR Facts.* Retrieved from http://www.nwcr.ws /Research/default.htm.

## Chapter 8

1. Burnette, J. L. & Finkel, E. J. (2012). Buffering against weight gain following dieting setbacks: An implicit theory intervention. *Journal of Experimental Psychology*, 48: 721–725. doi: 10.1016/j.jesp .2011.12.020. Retrieved from http://faculty.wcas.northwestern.edu/eli-finkel/documents/2012 _BurnetteFinkel_JESP.pdf.

2. Lally, P. et al. (2010). How are habits formed: Modelling habit formation in the real world. *European Journal of Social Psychology*, 40, 998–1009. doi: 10.1002/ejsp.674. Retrieved from http:// atlantaholisticmedicine.com/docs/How%20Habits%20are%20Formed.pdf.

## Chapter 9

1. Hall, K. D. et al. (2012). Energy balance and its components: Implications for body weight regulation. *The American Journal of Clinical Nutrition*, 95(4), 989–994. doi: 10.3945/ ajcn.112.036350. Retrieved from http://ajcn.nutrition.org/content/95/4/989.short.

2. Thomas, D. M. et al. (2014). Effect of dietary adherence on the body weight plateau: A mathematical model incorporating intermittent compliance with energy intake prescription. *American Journal of Clinical Nutrition*, 100(3), 787–795. doi: 10.3945/ ajcn.113.079822. Retrieved from http://ajcn.nutrition .org/content/100/3/787.short.

3. Camargo, A. et al. (2014). Dietary fat modifies lipid metabolism in the adipose tissue of metabolic syndrome patients. *Genes & Nutrition*, 9(4), 409. doi: 10.1007/s12263-014-0409-3. Retrieved from http://www.ncbi.nlm.nih.gov/pmc/articles/PMC4169067/; Bray, G. A. (2013). Energy and fructose from beverages sweetened with sugar or high-fructose corn syrup pose a health risk for some people. *Advanced Nutrition*, March 2013(4), 220–225. doi: 10.3945/ an.112.002816. Retrieved from http://advances.nutrition.org/content/4/2/220.full.pdf+html.

4. Digate Muth, N. (January 6, 2010). What should I eat before, during and after my workouts? *ACE Fit Life* online. Retrieved from https://www.acefitness.org/acefit/healthy-living-article/60/502/what -should-i-eat-before-during-and-after-my/.

## Chapter 10

1. Donnelly, J. E. et al. (2009). Appropriate Physical Activity Intervention Strategies for Weight Loss and Prevention of Weight Regain for Adults. *Journal of Medicine & Science in Sports & Exercise.* 4(12): 459-471. doi: 0.1249/MSS.0b013e3181949333. Retrieved from http://europepmc.org/abstract /med/19127177.

2. RunningUSA online. (2012). *2012 State of the Sport Part II: Running Industry Report.* Retrieved from http://www.runningusa.org/2012-state-of-sport-part-2?returnTo=annual-reports.

3. King, J. A. et al. (2010). The acute effects of swimming on appetite, food intake and plasma acylated ghrelin. *Journal of Obesity,* Volume 2011, Article ID 351628, 8 pages. doi:10.1155/2011/351628. Retrieved from http://www.hindawi.com/journals/jobe/2011/351628/.

4. Mitchell, W. K. et al. (2012). Sarcopenia, dynapenia, and the impact of advancing age on human skeletal muscle size and strength; a quantitative review. *Frontiers in Physiology,* 2012(3), 260. doi: 10.3389/fphys.2012.00260. Retrieved from http://www.ncbi.nlm.nih.gov/pmc/articles/PMC3429036/.

5. Egan, B. & Zierath, J. R. (2012). Exercise Metabolism and the Molecular Regulation of Skeletal Muscle Adaptation. *Cell Metabolism,* 17(2), 162–184. doi: 10.1016/j.cmet.2012.12.012. Retrieved from http://www.sciencedirect.com/science/article/pii/S1550413112005037.

6. Activity calorie calculations computed using the table from Harvard Health Publications online. (2004). Calories Burned in 30 Minutes for People of Three Different Weights. Retrieved from http://www.health.harvard.edu/newsweek/Calories-burned-in-30-minutes-of-leisure-and-routine-activities.htm.

## Chapter 11

1. Khoo, J. et al. (2010). Effects of a low-energy diet on sexual function and lower urinary Tract symptoms in obese men. *International Journal of Obesity,* 2010(34), 1396–1403. doi:10.1038/ijo.2010.76. Retrieved from http://www.nature.com/ijo/journal/v34/n9/abs/ijo201076a.html; Harvard School of Public Health online. Lipid and Nutrient Biology, Trafficking, Signaling and Chaperones in Metabolic Regulation. Retrieved from http://www.hsph.harvard.edu/gsh-lab/research/lipid-trafficking/.

2. Schaeffer, J. (October 2008). Taste better, live better: Using flavor to retrain palates and fill up on less. *Today's Dietician,* 10(10), 54. Retrieved from http://www.todaysdietitian.com/newarchives/092208p54.shtml; European Food Information Council online. (February 2011). Tastes differ: How taste preferences develop. Retrieved from http://www.eufic.org/article/en/health-and-lifestyle/food-choice/artid/how-taste-preferences-develop/.

3. European Food Information Council online. Tastes differ.

4. Mennella, J. A. et al. (2005). Genetic and environmental determinants of bitter perception and sweet preferences. *Pediatrics,* 115(2), e216-e222. doi: 10.1542/peds.2004-1582. Retrieved from http://pediatrics.aappublications.org/content/115/2/e216.abstract.

5. Spence, C. et al. (2010). Does food color influence taste and flavor perception in humans? *Chemosensory Perception,* 3(1), 68–84. doi: 10.1007/s12078-010-9067-z. Retrieved from http://psy.fgu.edu.tw/web/wlchou/general_psychology/class_pdf/Advanced%20Perceptual/2011/2011week4_ChengChung_paper.pdf.

6. Spence, C. & Deroy, O. (2013). On why music changes what (we think) we taste. *i-Perception,* 4(2), 137–140. doi:10.1068/i0577ic. Retrieved from http://www.ncbi.nlm.nih.gov/pmc/articles/PMC3677333/.

7. National Cancer Institute online. (Reviewed October 15, 2010). Chemicals in meat cooked at high temperatures and cancer risk. *NCI Fact Sheet.* Retrieved from http://www.cancer.gov/cancertopics/factsheet/Risk/cooked-meats.

8. Crowe, Aaron. (May 25, 2013). Good value, or no? Seven ways wholesale clubs make you spend more. *Christian Science Monitor* online. Retrieved from http://www.csmonitor.com/Business/Saving-Money/2013/0525/Good-value-or-no-Seven-ways-wholesale-clubs-make-you-spend-more.

9. Ledikwe, J. H. et al. (2005). Portion sizes and the obesity epidemic. *Journal of Nutrition*, 135(4), 905–909. Retrieved from http://jn.nutrition.org/content/135/4/905.full.pdf+html

10. Van Ittersum, K. & Wansink, B. (2012). Plate size and color suggestibility: The Delboeuf illusion's bias on serving and eating behavior. *Journal of Consumer Research*. 39(2): 215-228. doi:10.1086/662615. Retrieved from http://www.jstor.org/stable/10.1086/662615.

11. Ibid.

12. Stanhope, K. L. & Havel, P. J. (2008). Endocrine and metabolic effects of consuming beverages sweetened with fructose, glucose, sucrose, or high-fructose corn syrup. *American Journal of Clinical Nutrition*, 88(6), 1733S–1737S. doi: 10.3945/ajcn.2008.25825D http://ajcn.nutrition.org/content/88/6/1733S.long; Le, M. T. et al. (2012). Effects of high fructose corn syrup and sucrose on the pharmacokinetics of fructose and acute metabolic and hemodynamic responses in healthy subjects. *Metabolism*, 6(15), 641–651. doi: 10.1016/j.metabol.2011.09.013. Retrieved from http://www.ncbi.nlm.nih.gov/pmc/articles/PMC3306467/.

13. Fowler, S. P. et al. (2008). Fueling the obesity epidemic? Artificially sweetened beverage use and long-term weight gain. *Obesity*, 16(8): 1894–1900. doi: 10.1038/oby.2008.284. Retrieved from http://www.ncbi.nlm.nih.gov/pubmed/18535548.

14. Little, T. J. et al. (2014). Effects of varying the inter-meal interval on relationships between antral area, gut hormones and energy intake following a nutrient drink in healthy lean humans. *Physiology & Behavior*, 2014(135): 34–43. doi: 10.1016/j.physbeh.2014.05.040. Retrieved from http://www.ncbi.nlm.nih.gov/pubmed/24907689.

## Chapter 12

1. Brickman, P et al. (1978). Lottery winners and accident victims: Is happiness relative? *Journal of Personality and Social Psychology*, 38(8), 917–927. doi: 10.1037/0022-3514.36.8.917. Retrieved from http://www.researchgate.net/publication/22451114_Lottery_winners_and_accident_victims_is_happiness_relative.

2. Shlisky, J. D. et al. (2012). Partial sleep deprivation and energy balance in adults: An emerging issue for Consideration by Dietetics Practitioners. *Journal of the Academy of Nutrition and Dietetics*, 112(11), 1785–1797. doi: 10.1016/j.jand.2012.07.032. Retrieved from http://www.andjrnl.org/article/S2212-2672(12)01344-5/abstract.

3. Ibid.

4. Dallman, M. F. et al. (2003). Chronic stress and obesity: A new view of "comfort food." *Proceedings of the National Academy of Sciences*, September 30, 2003, 100(20), 11696–11701. doi: 10.1073/pnas.1934666100. Retrieved from http://www.ncbi.nlm.nih.gov/pmc/articles/PMC208820/.

5. Herring, M. P. et al. (2013). The effects of exercise training on anxiety. *American Journal of Lifestyle Medicine*. Published online 6 November 2013. doi: 10.1177/1559827613508542. Retrieved from http://ajl.sagepub.com/content/early/2013/11/06/1559827613508542.

## Chapter 13

1. Camps, S. G. et al. (2013). Weight loss, weight maintenance and adaptive thermogenesis. *American Journal of Clinical Nutrition*, 97(5), 990–994. doi: 10.3945/ ajcn.112.050310. Retrieved from http://ajcn.nutrition.org/content/97/5/990.full.

CPSIA information can be obtained at www.ICGtesting.com
Printed in the USA
BVOW07*1900230815

414653BV00019B/206/P